IMAGES
of America

ALBUQUERQUE DECO AND PUEBLO

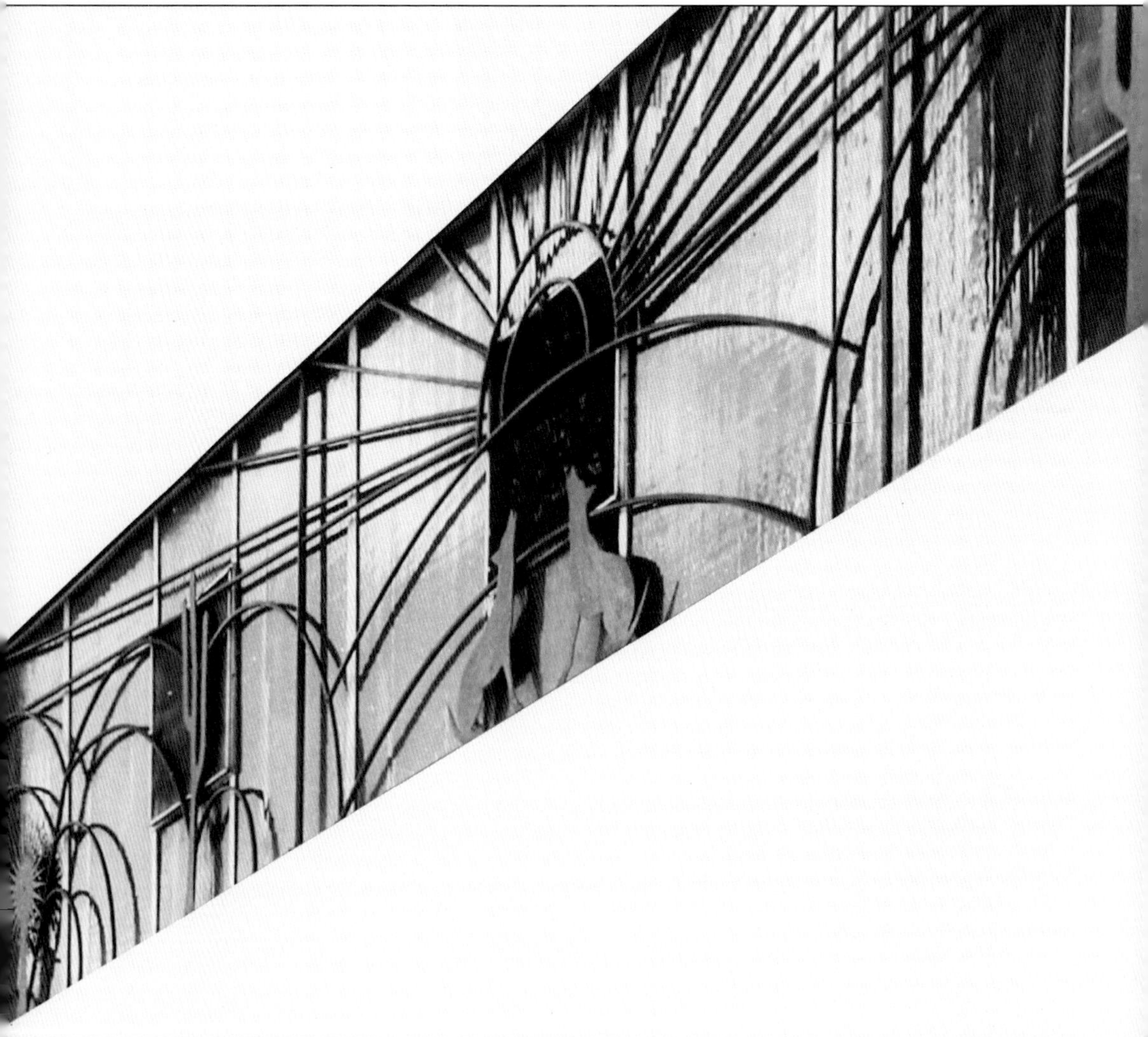

Pictured here is the Coyote Deco at Arrow Drug on Central Avenue in 1938. (See page 70.) (Courtesy of the Albuquerque Museum.)

On the Cover: Maisel's Indian Jewelry and Crafts, located at 510 Central Avenue SW, was designed by John Gaw Meem and opened in 1939. His client asked for "a strictly modern structure using where necessary Indian symbols." The mural created by Pueblo and Navajo artists unifies the entry. Cast aluminum molding surrounds the entrance door and evokes Native American designs. The cars are a 1948 Chevy Aero Coupe and a Plymouth. (Courtesy of the Albuquerque Museum.)

IMAGES
of America

ALBUQUERQUE DECO AND PUEBLO

Paul R. Secord

ARCADIA
PUBLISHING

ISBN 978-0-7385-9526-9

Published by Arcadia Publishing
Charleston, South Carolina

Printed in the United States of America

Library of Congress Control Number: 2011938564

For all general information, please contact Arcadia Publishing:
Telephone 843-853-2070
Fax 843-853-0044
E-mail sales@arcadiapublishing.com
For customer service and orders:
Toll-Free 1-888-313-2665

Visit us on the Internet at www.arcadiapublishing.com

To everyone who has helped keep the buildings in this book alive and remembered the ones that are gone.

Contents

ACKNOWLEDGMENTS

Many people made this book possible. Here is a partial list: my wife, Marcia, for her critical review and proofreading skills; the University of New Mexico (UNM), Center for Southwest Research staff and in particular Audra Bellmore, assistant professor and curator who unfailingly pointed me to the correct file and appeared minutes later with said file from the depths of the library; Skip and Jeanie Maisel for opening the Maisel files to me; Nancy Tucker for her selfless access to her amazing collection of Albuquerque images; Ed Boles, planner, City of Albuquerque Historic Preservation who literally showed me the town; Glenn Fye, photography curator of the Albuquerque City Museum; UNM professors Chris Wilson, who pointed me to several buildings I would not have found otherwise, and Ted Jojola, who opened my eyes to Isleta Pueblo and the Albuquerque Indian School; Larry McGowen and the federal marshals at the Federal Building who found some great images and opened the building to me; Darin Sand of Goodman Realty for everything I have on the Hilton Hotel; Larry Parker, manager of the Kimo Theater, for giving me the run of the Kimo; Mo Palmer and Mary Davis for their counsel; local architect Gene Dyer for the picture of his mother on her horse; Alma Pack of the Shaffer Hotel for opening the Shaffer files to me; Aimee Tang for information on Fremont's Fine Foods; my editor Lauren Hummer for her rapid response to all my questions and review of pictures and text—she kept it on schedule; and lastly to my friends Gordon Bronitsky for his marketing help; Ann Scheid for her insightful improvements to the text, proofreading, and encouragement; Paula Donahue and Jennifer Coile for their critical reading of the text; Steven Donahue for photographic printing; as well as Mayfield Marshall and Joe Mildenberger for their automobile identification skills.

Introduction

This book celebrates the cultural mixing of various Native American, Spanish, Mexican, Hispanic, and 19th- and 20th-century Anglo-American forms and motifs, which are unique to Albuquerque.

The discussion and pictures that follow focus on buildings, both in terms of their massing, i.e. geometric form, as well as their ornamentation. Five chapters look at a select group of building designs using contemporary images and focus on regional influences on the architecture of Albuquerque, New Mexico, during the first half of the 20th century. The purpose is to highlight local interpretations of distinctive "modern" architectural styles, with a special emphasis on Native American forms and motifs. The result shows how Albuquerque, and to a great extent the American Southwest, grappled with finding architecture suited to its unique physical and cultural landscape.

Native American building massing is locally referred to by the derisive term "low and brown." One- and two-story, flat-roofed residences are the ubiquitous style to this day. However, given the multistory nature of many prehistoric pueblos, as well as of the current form of Taos Pueblo, the Pueblo forms can also be tall, e.g. the Zimmerman Library at the University of New Mexico and the now lost Franciscan Hotel.

Native American decorative motifs are another matter. They can appear in a variety of contexts, as will be described later in this Introduction.

Building materials are given a cursory discussion in the descriptions that follow. They are only mentioned if there is something distinctive in their application to a particular building. While adobe is the material most often associated with the Southwest and continues to be used to this day, most of the structures presented here are made of brick, hollow tile, concrete, or are wood frame and stucco. Those structures that do have an adobe core have essentially all been covered with stucco.

Albuquerque, New Mexico, was and still is the principal crossroads for commerce and exemplifies the distinctive cultural traditions found in the American Southwest. In Albuquerque, there is room to embrace the multiculturalism of the Southwest, along with the incorporation of new trends and, for that matter, new cultures. Despite its geographic importance, Albuquerque at the time discussed in this book was a small place; the population was about only about 6,200 in 1900. In 1920, it was 15,200, and it was 26,600 in 1930. By 1940, it was still only 35,500. Substantial population did not come into the city until after the Second World War.

We cannot discuss Albuquerque's development without a brief digression to Santa Fe. Despite its importance as a political center, Santa Fe's population was roughly half that of Albuquerque's during the period under consideration. With statehood in 1912, Santa Fe began to re-create itself, primarily to promote tourism as a reflection of a near mythic past. The result was the ubiquitous "Santa Fe" style. A conscious effort was made to re-create, in fact to create, Santa Fe as a romantic and picturesque ancient city.

This re-creation followed the organizational structure of the then nationally prominent City Beautiful movement but with a mixing of indigenous design features, rather than the Beaux-Arts classicism typically associated with this movement. A comprehensive overview of the development of Santa Fe, from which much of this discussion is derived, is found in Chris Wilson's 1997 book *The Myth of Santa Fe.*

Mission-style forms, popular in Southern California, were rejected in Santa Fe in favor of what were seen as locally more "pure" Pueblo and simplified Spanish-Colonial forms of the Rio Grande Valley and immediate environs. The Mission style did find considerably greater expression in Albuquerque, given its adoption by the Santa Fe Railroad and Fred Harvey for his famous Harvey Houses, with Albuquerque's Alvarado Hotel complex being a major example, as well as the architectural theme for several large hospitals and sanatoriums.

Interestingly, the first expression of the Pueblo Revival idiom was not in Santa Fe but rather was a 1905 remodel of a building on the University of New Mexico campus in Albuquerque. Unfortunately, the idiom's leading proponent, Pres. William Tight, was dismissed in 1909, and the style was not revived on the campus until 1927.

Meanwhile, it was in Santa Fe where the new style was fully realized. The key arbiters were the staff of the Museum of New Mexico and School of American Archaeology—principally director Edgar Lee Hewett, photographer Jesse Nusbaum (later head of the rival Laboratory of Anthropology), illustrator Kenneth Chapman, and archaeologist Sylvanus Morley. Architects Isaac Rapp and in particular John Gaw Meem were to refine and realize the Santa Fe style as a coherent architectural movement.

Meem is an especially important figure. His focus was not to re-create the past but rather to successfully blend traditional forms and materials with modern requirements. Meem was for many years the chief architect for the University of New Mexico in Albuquerque, where he saw realized the execution of some of his most innovative and distinctive buildings.

While Albuquerque, as the commercial and transportation hub of the region also embraced Santa Fe's celebration of the past, Albuquerque also looked to modernism. Meem's atypical design for Maisel's Indian Store is one of the centerpieces of this book. And the design for the unrealized 1937 Sims Building, a multistory Art Deco office structure, may surprise those who associate Meem solely with the Santa Fe style.

Modernism was the defining architectural and applied arts style from the first quarter of the 20th century until World War II. During this period, being modern took a number of routes that typically attempted to divest itself from references to the past, i.e. rejecting Victorian ornament, as well as historic references of the Arts and Crafts movement that was itself a reaction to Victorianism.

Modern meant steel, cast concrete, and glass buildings. It meant a lack of ornamentation, and when ornamentation was embraced, the ornaments were not instantly recognizable as a reflection of a classical or medieval past. Modernism unapologetically embraced the age of the machine, most dramatically expressed in the Streamline Moderne movement of the 1930s.

What we now call Art Deco is a term coined in 1968 by Bevis Hillier to articulate a worldwide reaction to the 1925 Paris L'Exposition Internationale des Artes Decoratifs et Industriels Modernes. It refers as much to a characteristic ornamentation vocabulary as it does to building massing. Zigzag Moderne was associated with the 1920s and lent itself especially well to Native American motifs, as will be seen in Albuquerque's Pueblo Deco buildings, and to commercial facades, such as 616 Central Avenue (Fremont's Fine Foods) and the Skinner Building.

The 1930s Streamline Moderne is exemplified by several residences, such as the Kelvin House and Lembke House. While Albuquerque's later response to the modern in some cases resulted in characteristic International-style buildings, the Clyde Odin House is a fairly rare residence in this style (although there are a handful of other examples in Albuquerque).

The Moderne movement took a unique regional and sometimes bizarre turn that was centered in Albuquerque. An effort was made to apply Art Deco style, i.e. Moderne, to the architecture and motifs of varied Native American populations, along with those of the Spanish-speaking population. The initial flowering of this effort was by then established as Santa Fe style. The

1920s and 1930s result was Pueblo Deco, a descriptive term apparently coined in 1984 by Marcus Whiffen and Carla Breeze and used in the title of their book, *Pueblo Déco: The Architecture of the Southwest.*

The word *pueblo*, as it is commonly used in the Southwest, refers specifically to the term the Spanish used to describe four linguistically distinct Native American peoples found in New Mexico and northern Arizona. Pueblo is the Spanish word for village, and these Native Americans led an agricultural life that was centered in permanent multistoried villages.

Pueblo Deco, as an architectural term now in common parlance in the region, has a much broader range of influences than those exhibited by the Pueblo Indians. It is a highly eclectic style rarely restricted to one cultural tradition. Most buildings in the style exhibit some combination of motifs that include the following: (1) Pueblo pottery, ceremonies, rock art, and jewelry, (2) Navajo rugs, ceremonies, and jewelry, (3) Anglo ideas of what is "Indian," usually derived from Plains Indians, (4) influences of the Spanish-speaking populations of the Southwest, referring to Spanish, Mexican, or Hispanic, and (5) the wild west cowboys.

Wilson's book, *The Myth of Santa Fe*, includes a chapter interlude entitled, "Coyote Consciousness." He uses the metaphor of the coyote, primarily as expressed in various Native American stories, to describe the cultural complexity and ambiguity of the Southwest. The early-20th-century tourist promotional myth of three distinct cultures living in harmony—Indian, Spanish, and white, now transmogrified into Native Americans, Hispanics, and Anglo—is a much more varied with not necessarily harmonious associations. Rather it is, and continues to be, a process of blending, differentiation, and accommodation.

When cultural myths collided with modern architectural movements in the 1920s and 1930s, the result was not just Pueblo Deco, I believe it was "Coyote Deco." At its most sophisticated, the result is the Albuquerque Indian Hospital and Maisel's Indian store entrance. At its most playful and campy, the result is the Shaffer Hotel and the Kimo Theater. These buildings retain their original use and have been restored to their former glory. In 2011, a re-creation of the Kimo's original sign was installed.

Unfortunately, the term coyote has now taken on a pejorative connotation, given its association with human trafficking across the Mexican border. Howling coyotes, which were once common as tourist items, have been replaced by the Native American rock art figure Kokopelli, the hunchback flute player.

As noted, Native American themes are given particular attention in this book. They are no better expressed than on the 17 murals fronting Maisel's Indian Jewelry and Crafts, which is located at 510 Central Avenue SW. These murals, painted in 1937, are by mostly Native American art students who all became seminal members of the now thriving Native American art movement. Here is a building designed by John Gaw Meem, with cast aluminum Art Deco molding and a black Carrara glass front, coupled with the most traditional of Navajo, Apache, and Pueblo images done in a style that is instantly evocative of the 1930s. Because of their importance, and the fact that they are an integral part of the subject building, they are presented here, apparently for the first time in their entirety, as a final chapter. For more background on Native American paintings, see *Indian Painters and White Patrons* by J.J. Brody (University of New Mexico Press, 1971).

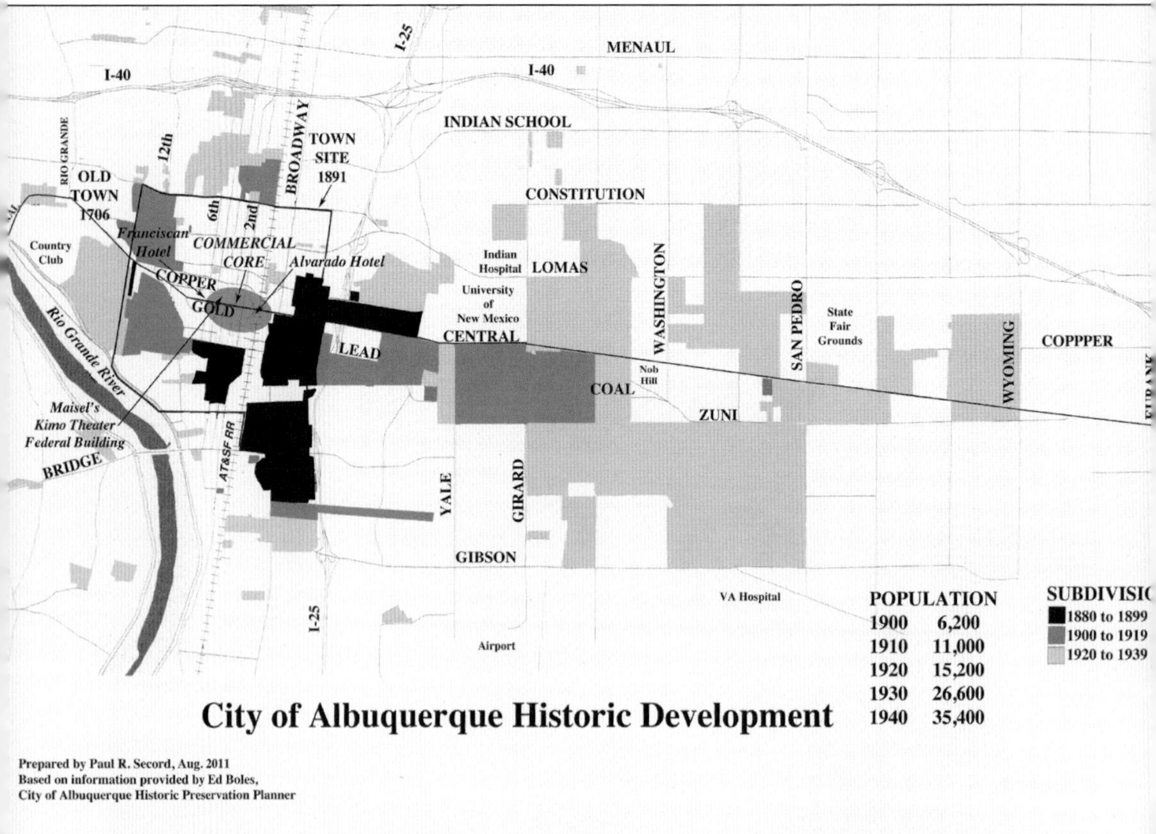

This map was prepared by the author using information provided by the Albuquerque City Planning Department. It illustrates residential subdivisions through 1939 and indicates the location of key Albuquerque buildings and streets covered in this book.

One

Building Styles

The chapters that follow are organized by building type rather than by architectural style, i.e. public buildings, commercial buildings, hotels, hospitals and sanatoriums, and residential structures. As noted previously, the final chapter presents pictures of all the Native American murals that form an integral part of the front facade of Maisel's Indian Jewelry and Crafts store. Please note: motels are not included since they are well covered in Arcadia Publishing's *Route 66 in New Mexico.*

This book is not intended as a guidebook or comprehensive survey. Rather it looks at buildings that were viewed as modern at the time of their construction, which at the same time harmonized with the varied cultural traditions of the region's past. The result is a sample skewed towards structures that have Native American influences, that are unique, and/or that have already been determined to be locally or regionally significant.

The first chapter is a generalized style guide that serves to define and illustrate key diagnostic building features found in this book. The style descriptions are derived, with some modification, from architectural identification guidelines used by City of Albuquerque and State of New Mexico historic preservation planners.

A number of the architectural styles that are distinctive of the mid- to late 19th century are found in Albuquerque and carried on into the first quarter of the 20th century. These styles are, for the most part, ubiquitous throughout the United States and typically look to European antecedents. They include Queen Anne houses with steeply pitched hipped roofs and porches and occasionally Italianate buildings with their ornate heavy brackets under wide eaves as well as the French-derived Mansard (Second Empire) style houses with their double-pitched hipped roofs. Colonial Revival, Neoclassic, American Foursquare, and Bungalow (Craftsman) styles are also found. In addition, various European Revival styles are especially common in residential architecture from the 1920s to 1930s, including Spanish Eclectic or Mediterranean-style buildings with red-tiled roofs. Except for a few dominant or highly distinctive examples, these styles are not represented here. The following pages present examples of the principal styles that are included.

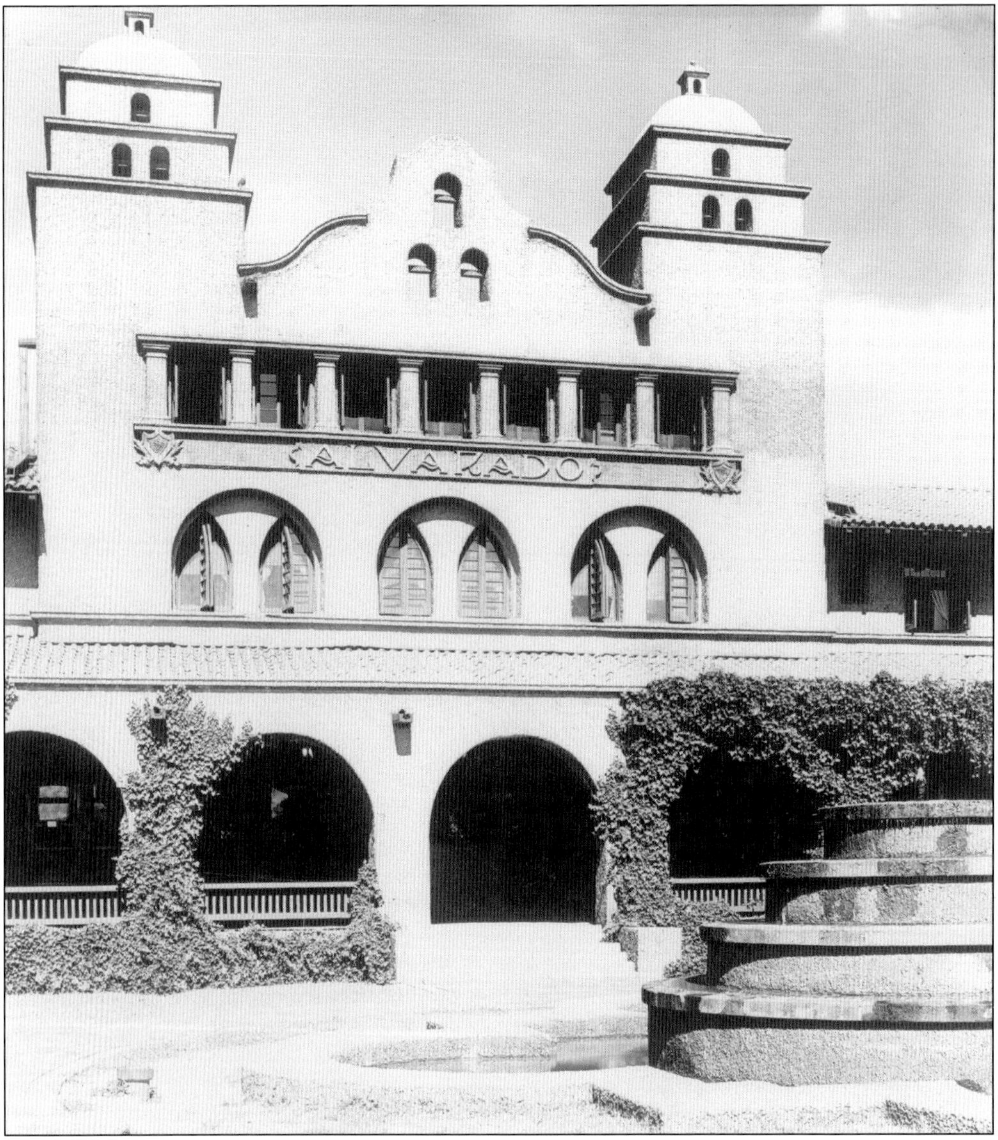

The Alvarado Hotel, designed in the California Mission Revival style (1900–1930), was built in 1902 and demolished in 1970. The diagnostic features are plain walls, arched openings, low-pitched tile roofs, paired bell towers, occasional use of small domes, and what detailing does occur relates to Spanish, Moorish, and Islamic forms. This style especially came to national attention following its use for the California Building at the 1893 Chicago World's Fair. It presents a romanticized interpretation of Spanish Colonial Mission architecture and was popular for a wide range of building types. By 1900, it had became the preferred style for railroad terminals and the famous Harvey Houses, of which this building is an example. Use of Mission Revival architecture in New Mexico represents a romanticized attempt at finding a style suited to the southwestern environment, while its adoption by the railroad ensured substantial commissions from the outset. In Albuquerque, it was especially popular for hospitals, sanatoriums, and schools. The 1915 Panama-California Exposition in San Diego, California, was especially influential in popularizing this architectural style to a national audience as well as the Pueblo Revival style that ultimately became the ubiquitous New Mexico regional style. (Courtesy of Nancy Tucker.)

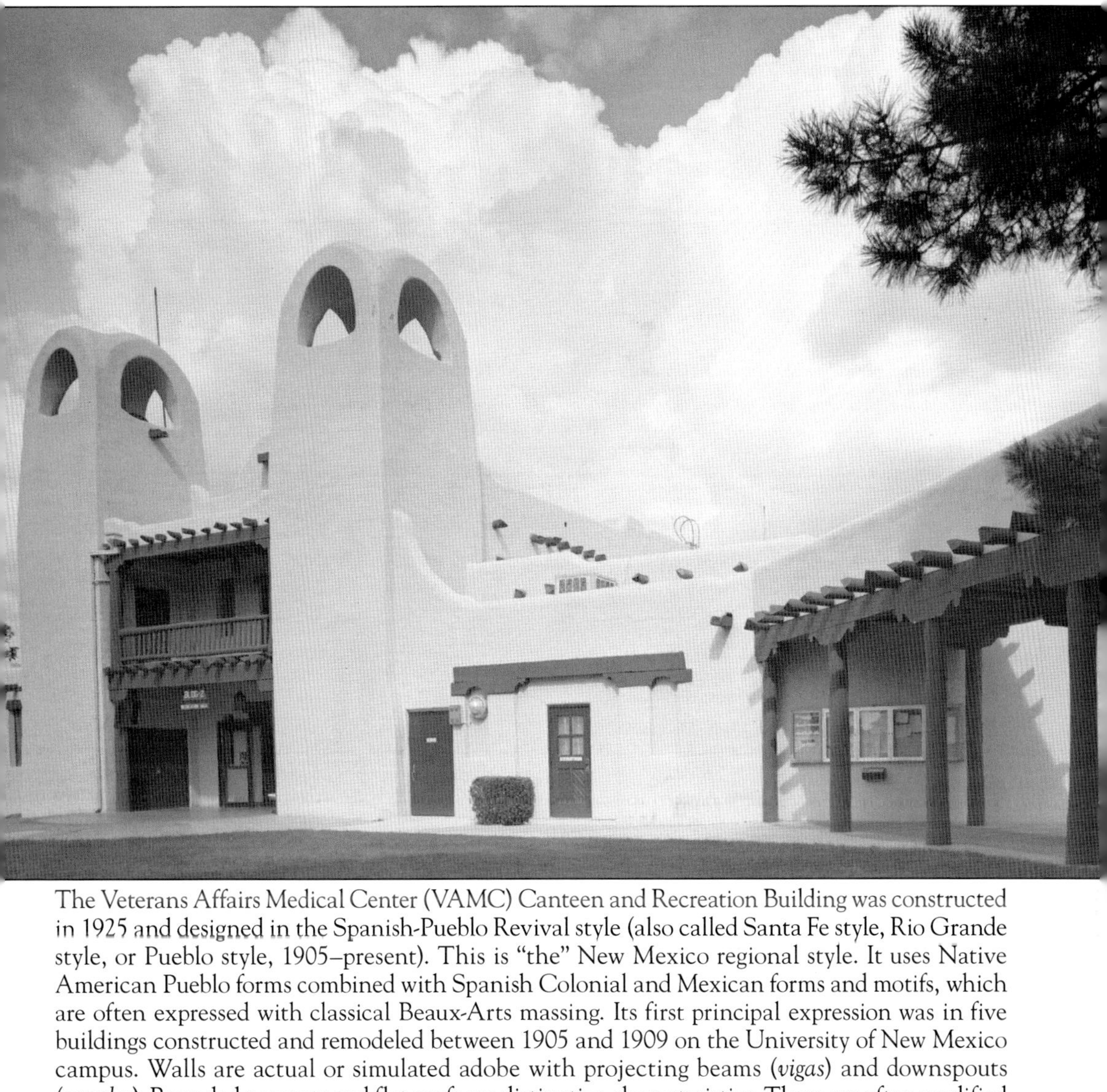

The Veterans Affairs Medical Center (VAMC) Canteen and Recreation Building was constructed in 1925 and designed in the Spanish-Pueblo Revival style (also called Santa Fe style, Rio Grande style, or Pueblo style, 1905–present). This is "the" New Mexico regional style. It uses Native American Pueblo forms combined with Spanish Colonial and Mexican forms and motifs, which are often expressed with classical Beaux-Arts massing. Its first principal expression was in five buildings constructed and remodeled between 1905 and 1909 on the University of New Mexico campus. Walls are actual or simulated adobe with projecting beams (*vigas*) and downspouts (*canales*). Rounded parapets and flat roofs are distinctive characteristics. There are often modified church fronts, as with this example, as well as round columns topped by corbel brackets supporting front esplanades and porches. The style has seen various distinctive phases and reaches its most sophisticated expression in the work of architect John Gaw Meem, who lived in Albuquerque and who was for many years the chief architect for the University of New Mexico. (Courtesy of the National Archives, Historic American Building Survey.)

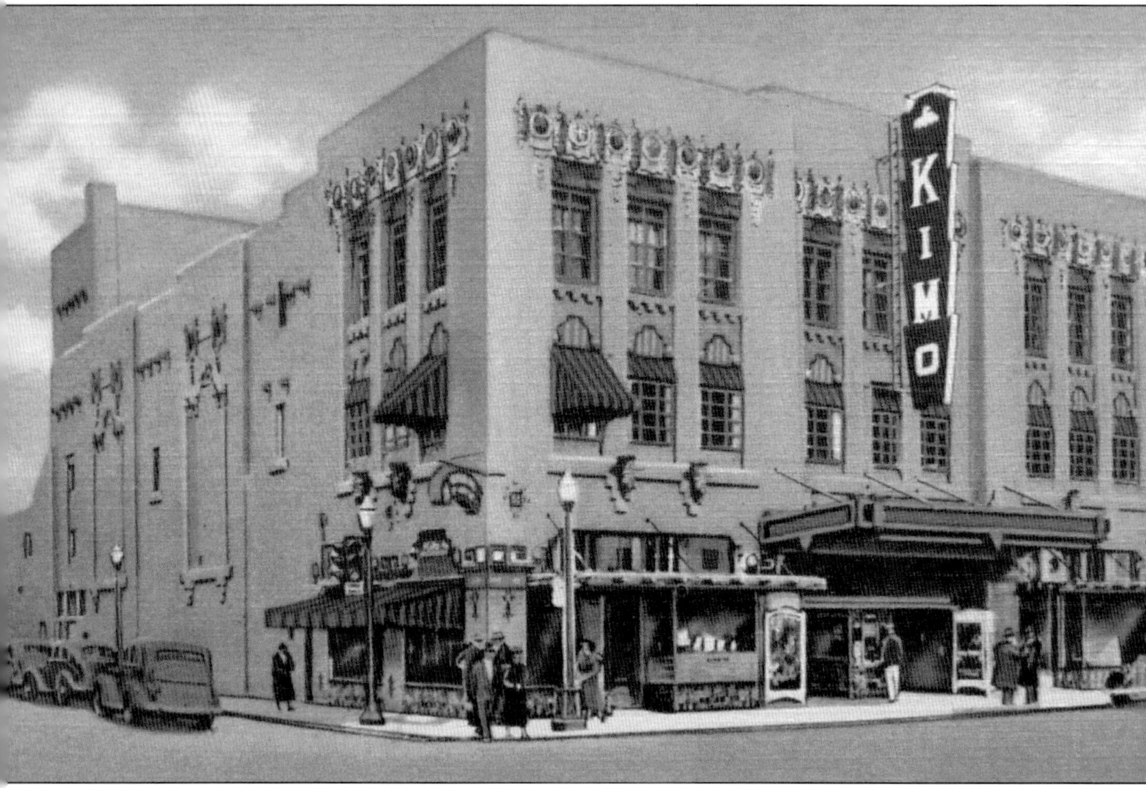

The Kimo Theater was built in 1927 and its design typifies the Pueblo Deco style (1930–1945). As noted in the Introduction, the Art Deco movement of the 1920s and 1930s took an individualistic turn in Albuquerque. The key features of this variant style are applied ornamentation that incorporates Native American motifs with typical geometric Art Deco patterns, primarily of the 1920s. Decorating the tops of the theater's third-story windows are colorful Pueblo shields, executed in geometric tile work. There are also Indian symbols painted on the building. (Courtesy of Nancy Tucker.)

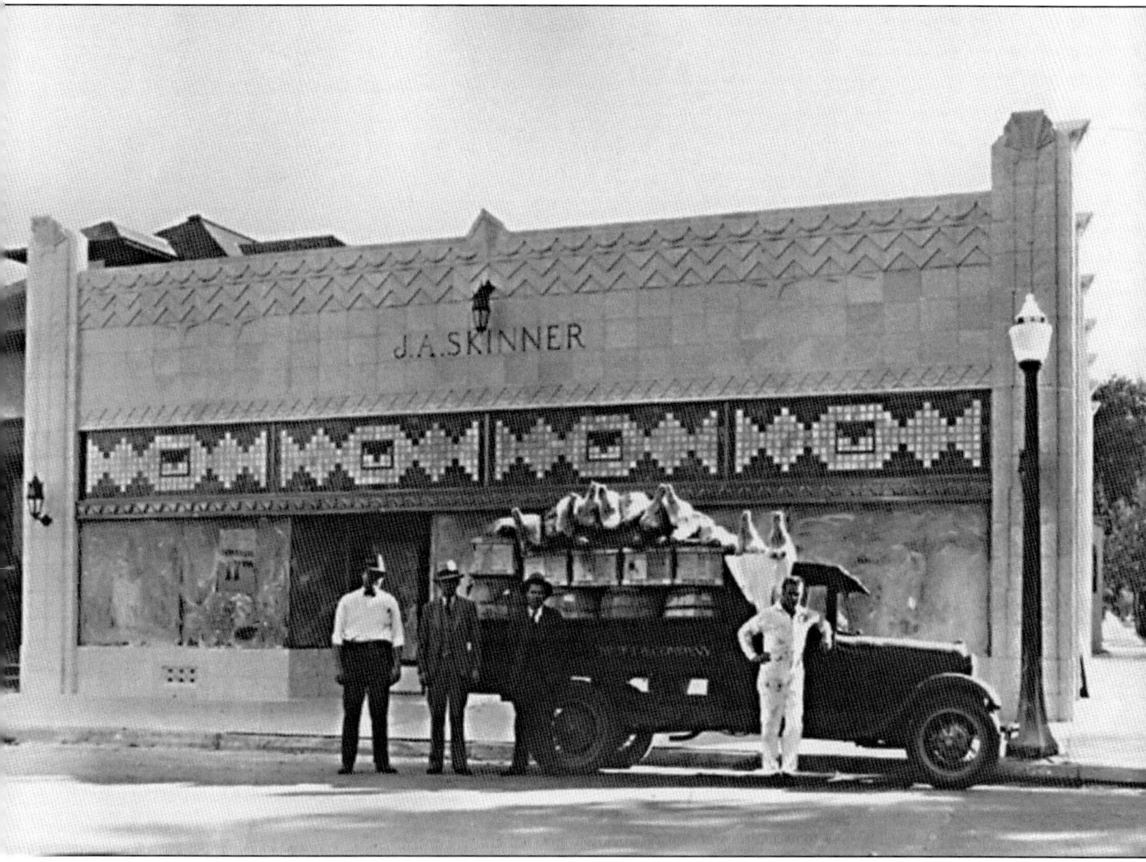

The Skinner Building (1931) was constructed in the Zigzag Art Deco style (1920–1941). This is the 1920s expression of the Moderne or Art Deco movement. It is derived from classically inspired designs of the 1910s and early 1920s. Characteristic ornamentation includes zigzags, chevrons, sunbursts, spirals, and stylized plant and animal motifs. Native American designs are especially well suited to these forms and often appear on buildings of this period in Albuquerque. (Courtesy of the Museum of Albuquerque.)

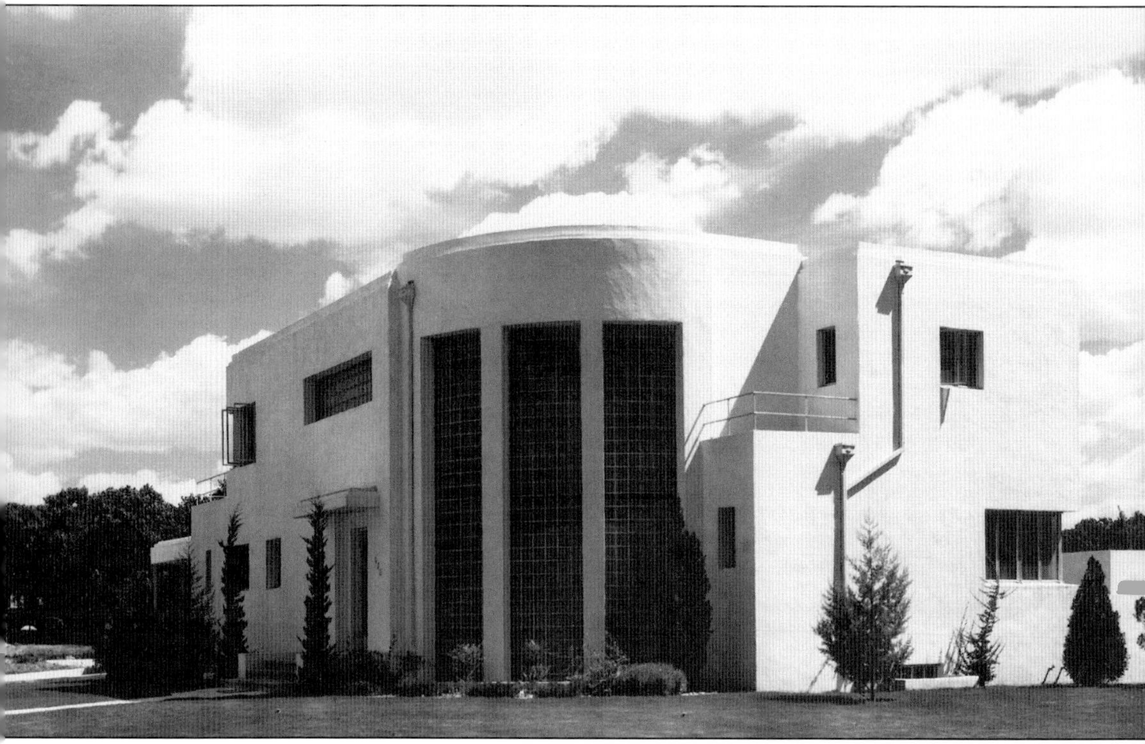

The Lembke House (1937) was built in a Streamline Moderne style (Moderne, Depression Moderne, 1930–1950). Here is the 1930s rendering of Art Deco. Key features to look for are rounded corners with horizontal bands, often in aluminum and glass bricks; projecting wings and lighthouse towers are common. (Courtesy of the Museum of Albuquerque.)

Two

Public Buildings

The survey of Albuquerque architecture opens with public buildings. By 1900, Albuquerque was the transportation, medical, and educational center of the state, a position that was enhanced by New Mexico statehood in 1912. Santa Fe retained its importance as the governmental center, and the home to the state prison. The railroad, hospitals, sanatoriums, and schools provided Albuquerque with an employment base and architectural focus that Santa Fe lacked. The Atchison, Topeka &Santa Fe (AT&SF) train station and Fred Harvey's Alvarado Hotel (1901–1904) were the largest California Mission-style buildings in the region. The University of New Mexico (UNM) flirted with Pueblo Revival architecture for several buildings between 1905 and 1909. After a gap of over 15 years, the Spanish-Pueblo Revival became the exclusive architectural style of UNM for most of the 20th century after John Gaw Meem became campus architect. The Mission style initially had a strong presence in Albuquerque. Its use in New Mexico is clearly derived from romantic notions popularized by the California mission preservation movement spearheaded by Charles Lummis and George Wharton James. Ironically, while New Mexican missions predate California missions by 150 years, some remodeled in later centuries were stripped of their Baroque architectural features. Such features are associated with California missions. Many of these early buildings were either abandoned or in some state of ruin long before 1900. The Isleta Pueblo Church (1613) was one of the few New Mexico missions to retain some of its "mission" look into the 19th century. Native American influences in public architecture are especially well expressed in the ornamentation of Albuquerque's 1930 Federal Building. Also, in 1931, the Albuquerque Indian School Employee Dormitory and Club was constructed in the Mission style, the only building designed by a Native American in this survey.

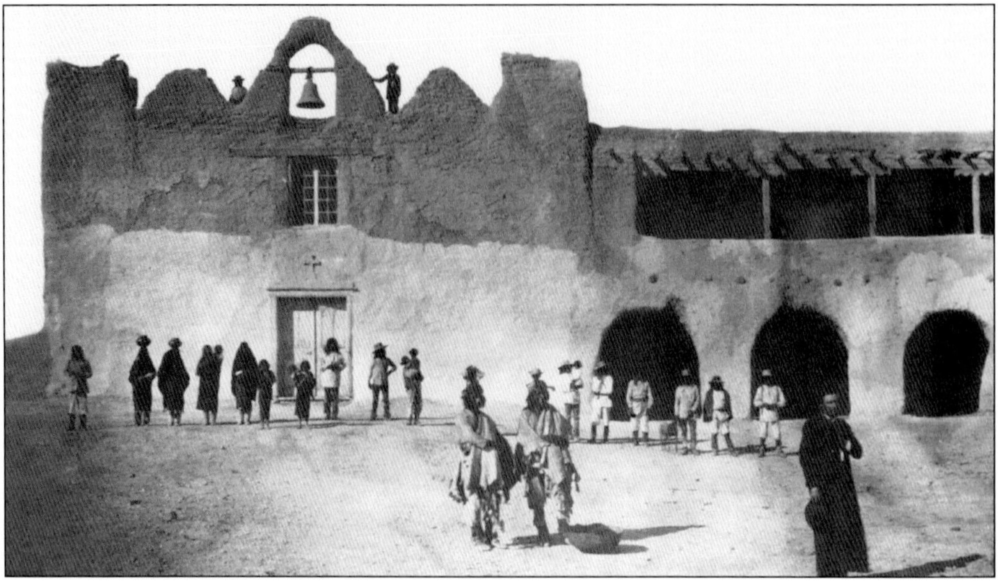

The Isleta Pueblo Church is an allegory for the Spanish-Pueblo Revival part of the story. The church was founded in 1613 and rebuilt in 1716, with many later changes. Above is the church in 1867, one of the earliest photographs in New Mexico. The bell arch over the front door was added in 1776, while the rare *convento* arches are earlier. The arches were gone before 1900. A 1923 remodel by Fr. Anton Docher saw unfortunate additions, including a high-pitched roof, elaborate wooden corner spires, and an odd front porch. In 1962, a more appropriate remodel was carried out. Below is a postcard from 1960s. This is today's church, with a flat roof, bell in each of the two centered mission arches, and tile roofed corner towers. Is this Mission Restoration or Mission Revival style? (Above, courtesy of Southern Methodist University; below, author's collection.)

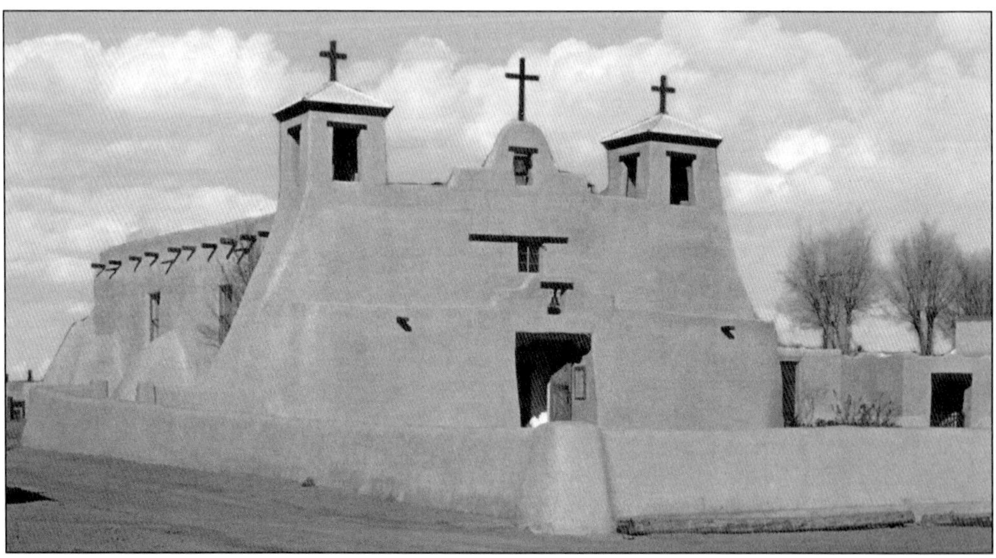

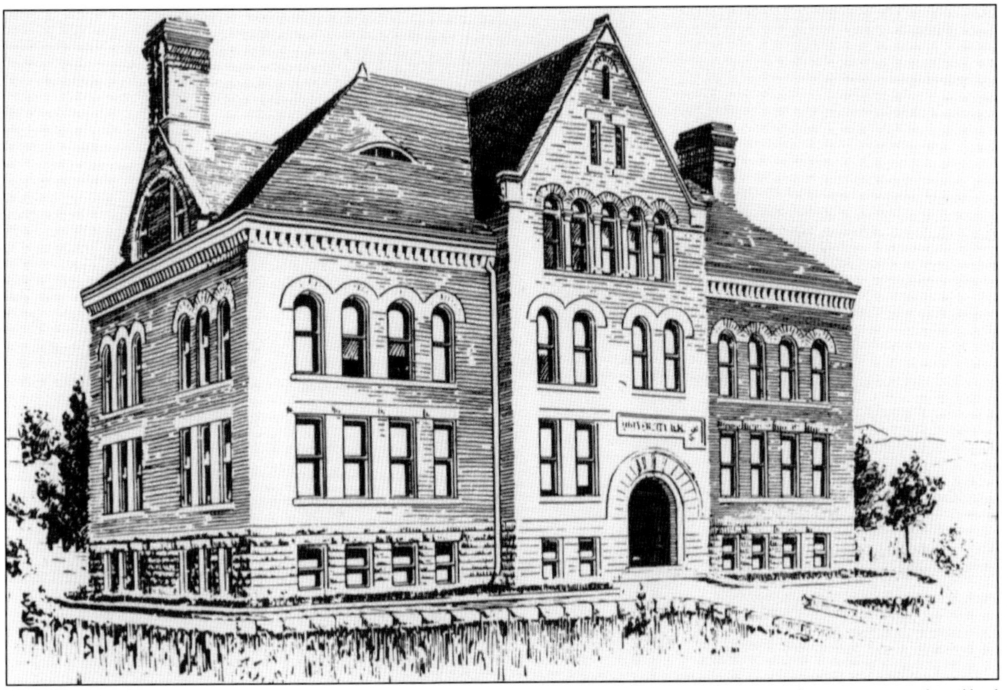

The first building on the University of New Mexico campus was constructed in 1892 and called the Main Building. It was designed by Jesse M. Wheelock as a redbrick Richardsonian Romanesque structure. In 1908, it was dramatically remodeled in the Pueblo Revival style. University president George Tight and campus architect E.B. Cristy designed the remodel. There are reports that Mary Coulter of Harvey House fame was also involved with the design. In 1936, the Main Building was renamed Hodgin Hall, and it serves as the UNM Alumni House today. Between 1905 and 1910, Pueblo Revival became the campus style, although only about a half dozen of such buildings were constructed during that early period. (Both, courtesy of UNM CSWR Hodgin Photograph Collection.)

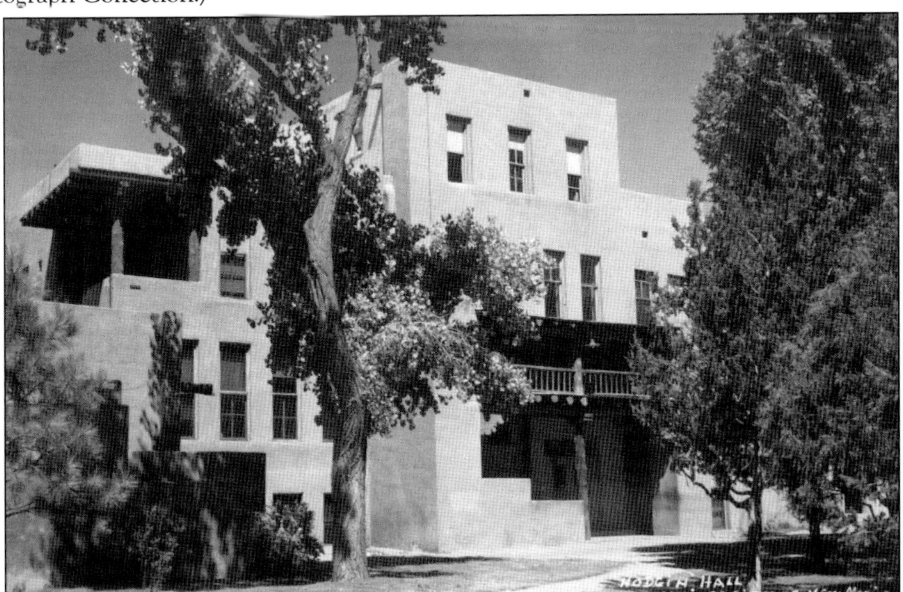

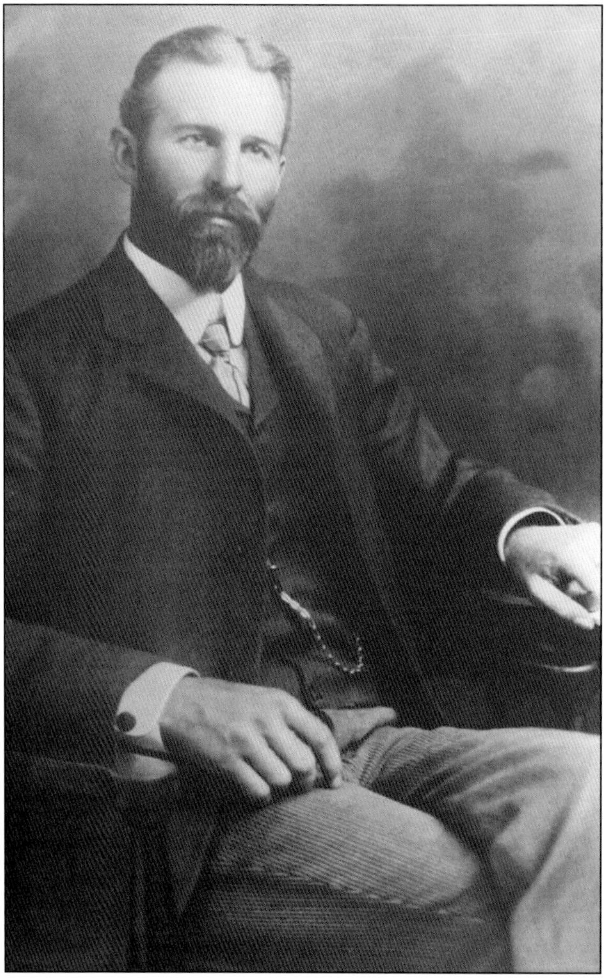

William George Tight (1858–1910), the third president of UNM, helped build the house he lived in, which is seen below about 1906. It was demolished in 1964. Tight and university architect Edward Buxton Cristy (1860–1934) invented Pueblo Revival architecture. Tight reasoned that university life was "communal and similar to pueblo life in its living arrangements and ceremonial requirements." He thought the university should become the "Pueblo on the Mesa." Tight's vision was generally well received, including articles in the national architectural trade press. Note that UNM's Pueblo architecture predates the 1910–1912 renovation of the Santa Fe Palace of the Governors. Unfortunately, charges that Tight overstepped his authority in firing two faculty members and, though divorced, carried on a dalliance with a single female faculty member forced his resignation in 1909. This ended UNM's Pueblo-style architecture until the mid-1920s. (Both, courtesy of UNM CSWR Campus Archives.)

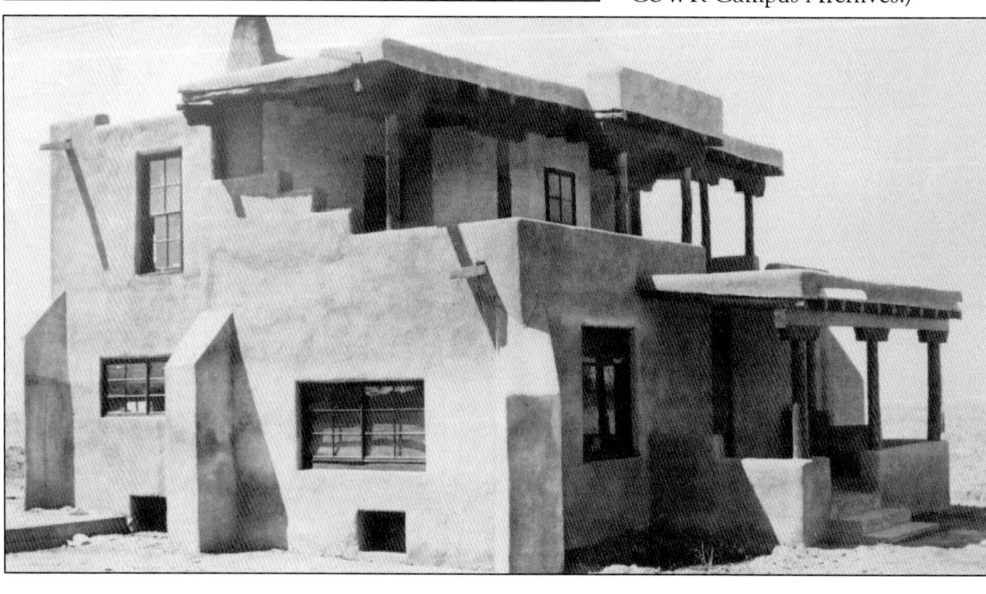

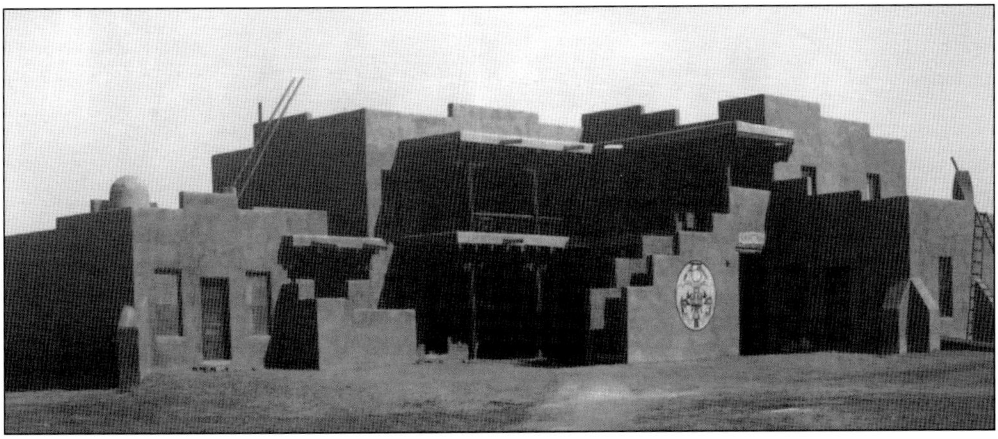

Pictured here is the full flowering of Tight's vision, the first dorms on the UNM campus, both built in 1906. At the top is Hokona ("maiden butterfly") Hall, and at the bottom is Kwataka ("man eagle") Hall. These residences were furnished with Navajo rugs and rustic furniture. They had electric lights as well as solar water heating systems concealed on the roof as Spanish-style beehive ovens called *hornos*. The exterior walls featured large designs inspired by Hopi pottery and painted by Tight and an English teacher, Ethel Hickey. (Both, courtesy of Nancy Tucker.)

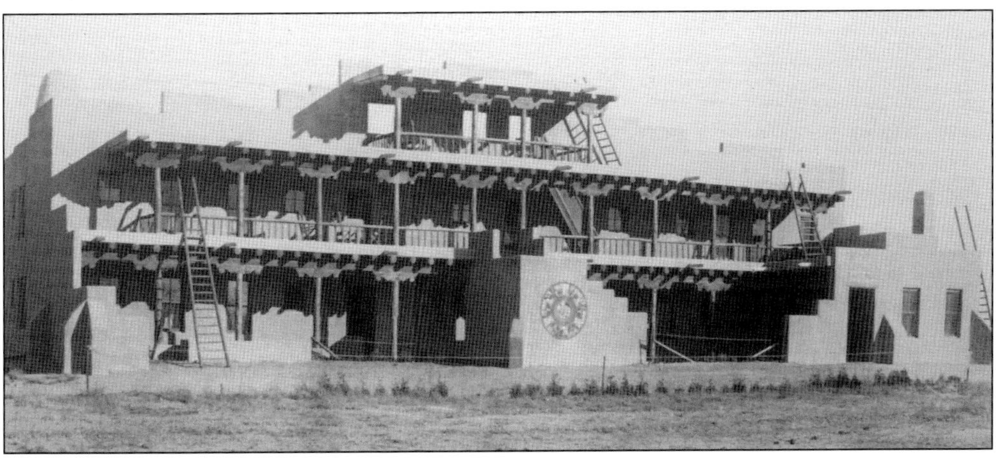

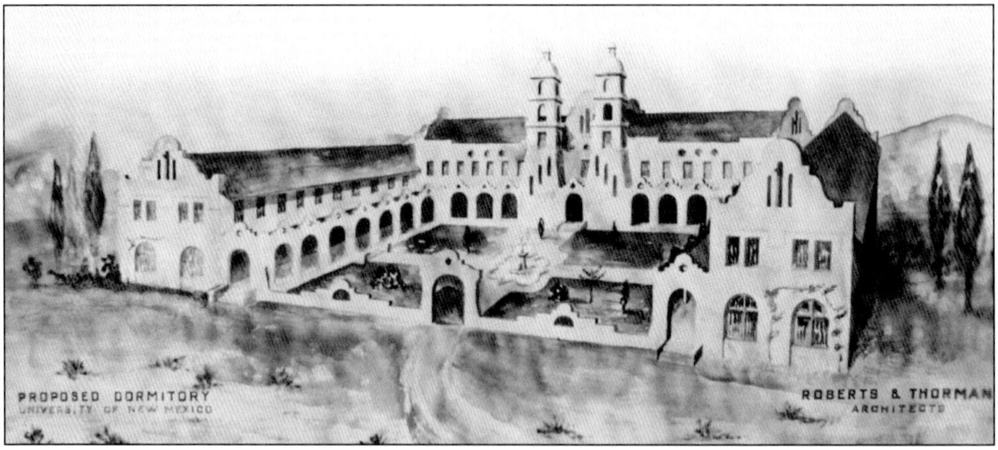

The local Albuquerque architectural firm of Roberts & Thorman prepared this design for an unrealized Mission Revival–style UNM dormitory. The firm was only active between 1909 and 1910, after which O.H. Thorman moved to El Paso, Texas, where he had a long and productive career. Perhaps inspired by the Alvarado Hotel, this rejected design appears to be dated after President Tight's resignation. (Courtesy of UNM CSWR Hodgin Photograph Collection.)

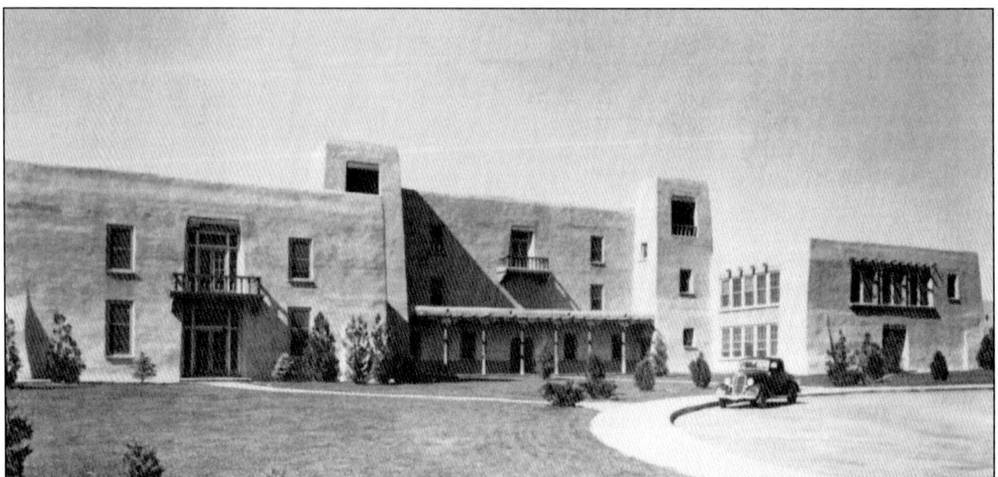

UNM architecture was ultimately defined by John Gaw Meem (1894–1983), the "campus architect" from 1934 to 1956. He was instrumental in articulating and refining the Spanish-Pueblo Revival style. His first campus building in 1934, a multipurpose structure, was named Scholes Hall in 1969 and was inspired by early Spanish mission churches in New Mexico. Its twin towers were reminiscent of San Esteban del Rey church at Acoma Pueblo. Scholes Hall has wonderful Art Deco interior detailing. (Courtesy of Nancy Tucker.)

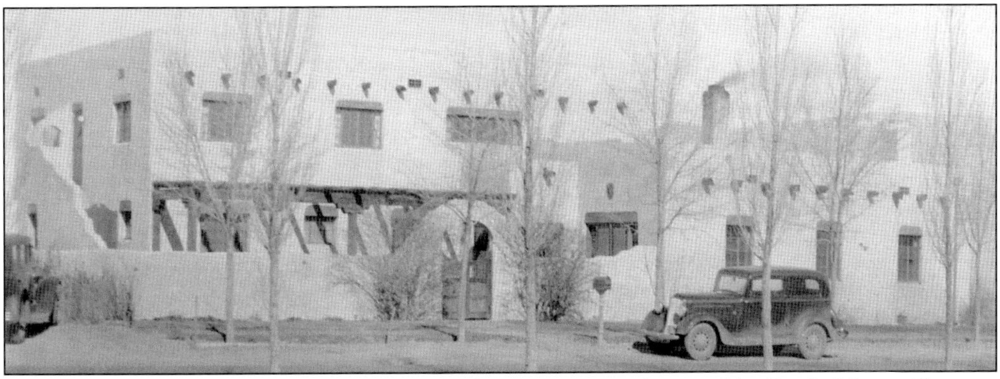

The Alpha Chi Omega Sorority House, built in 1930, was designed by Buela Nixon Fleming (1904–1980). She was one of the first, if not the first, female architects to practice in Albuquerque. Fleming, a native New Mexican, designed a number of residences in Albuquerque during the 1930s and 1940s. This Spanish-Pueblo Revival residential structure exhibits many of the characteristic features of the style. The building was acquired by the university in 1968 and is used as office space today. (Courtesy of Nancy Tucker.)

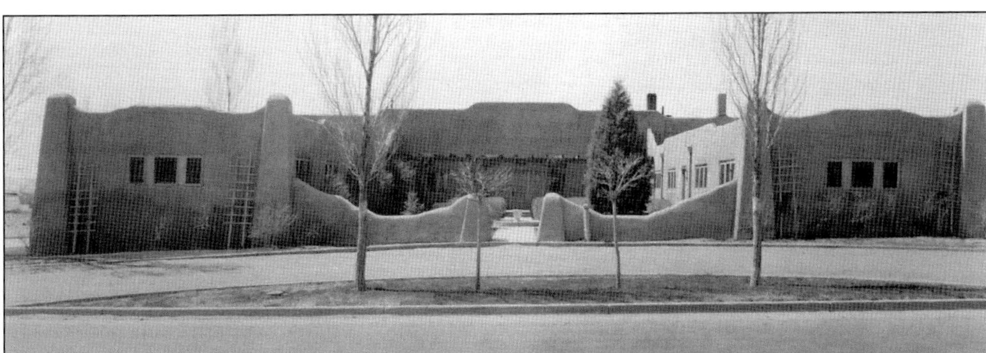

Kappa Sigma Fraternity occupied this house, which was built in 1926. The design, by professor Charles T. Coan, chairman of the UNM History Department at the time, is a fine example of Spanish-Pueblo Revival. Compare it with Meem's Scholes Hall. Sadly, this building was condemned and demolished in 1984. (Courtesy of Nancy Tucker.)

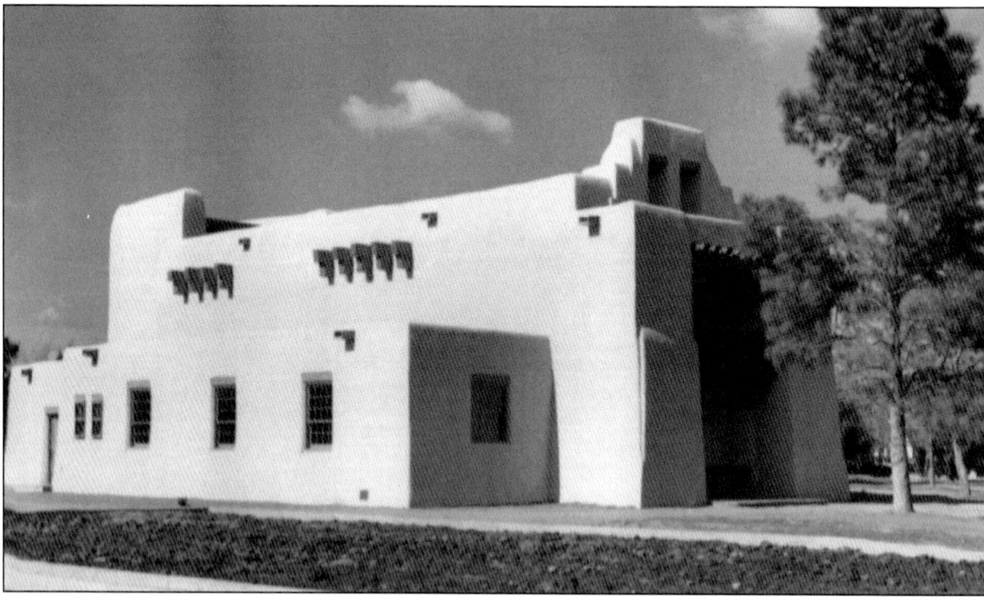

The Alumni Memorial Chapel was designed by Meem, Holien, Buckley, and Associates in 1954 and built in 1962. It was Meem's last building on the campus and is next to Scholes Hall, his first campus structure. It is an excellent example of John Gaw Meem's religious structures, designed in Spanish-Pueblo Revival style, based on traditional New Mexico Pueblo and village church architecture. It echoes many earlier Meem-designed chapels. (Courtesy of Nancy Tucker.)

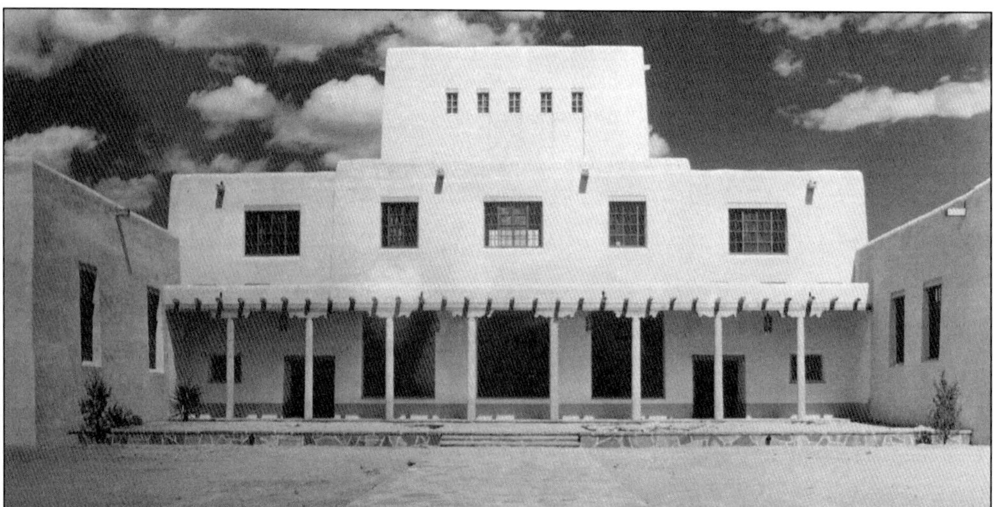

University Library, dedicated in 1938, was named in 1961 for James Zimmerman, UNM president from 1928 to 1944. It is considered John Gaw Meem's finest Pueblo-style design. Local Native American and Hispanic artisans handcrafted the structure's wood and metalwork, funded by the Public Works Administration (PWA) and Works Progress Administration (WPA). The interior reading rooms and main corridor are in original condition, with furniture, lighting, and other decorative fittings designed by Meem. (Courtesy of Nancy Tucker.)

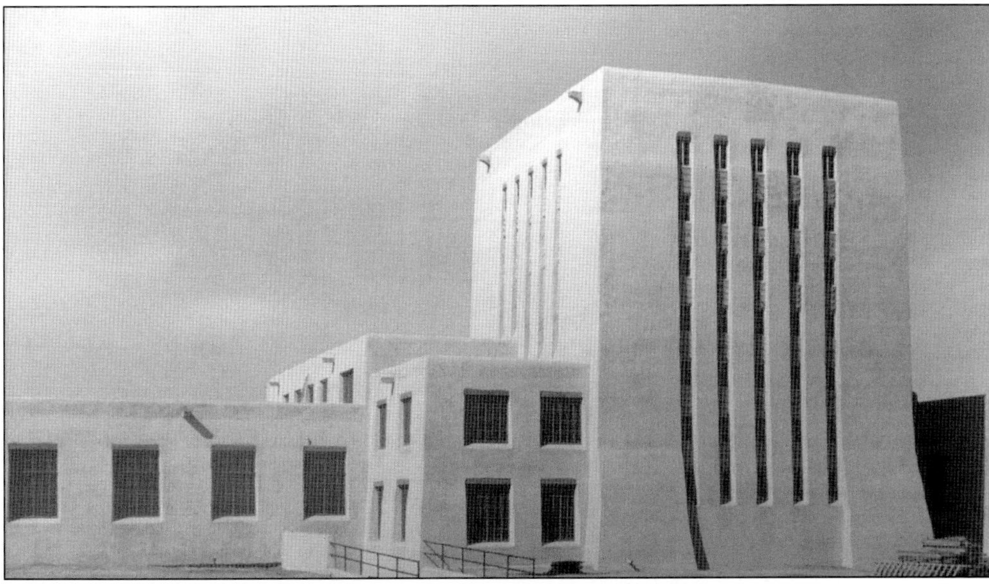

Pictured here are University (Zimmerman) Library under construction in the fall of 1937 and the reference and periodicals desk. The tall book storage tower was designed to be the focal point of the campus. Dorothy Hughes writes in *Pueblo on the Mesa*, "The towering new building was designed and guarded in its architectural authenticity by John Gaw Meem . . . Colonnaded portals, wrought iron grilles, high wood ceilings with carved *vigas* and *savions*, authentic beams and corbels, diagonal *latillas*, carved doors and cases, Mexican tin lighting fixtures hand-made by native craftsmen . . . all is beautifully created in the Spanish and Indian tradition." (Both, courtesy of Nancy Tucker.)

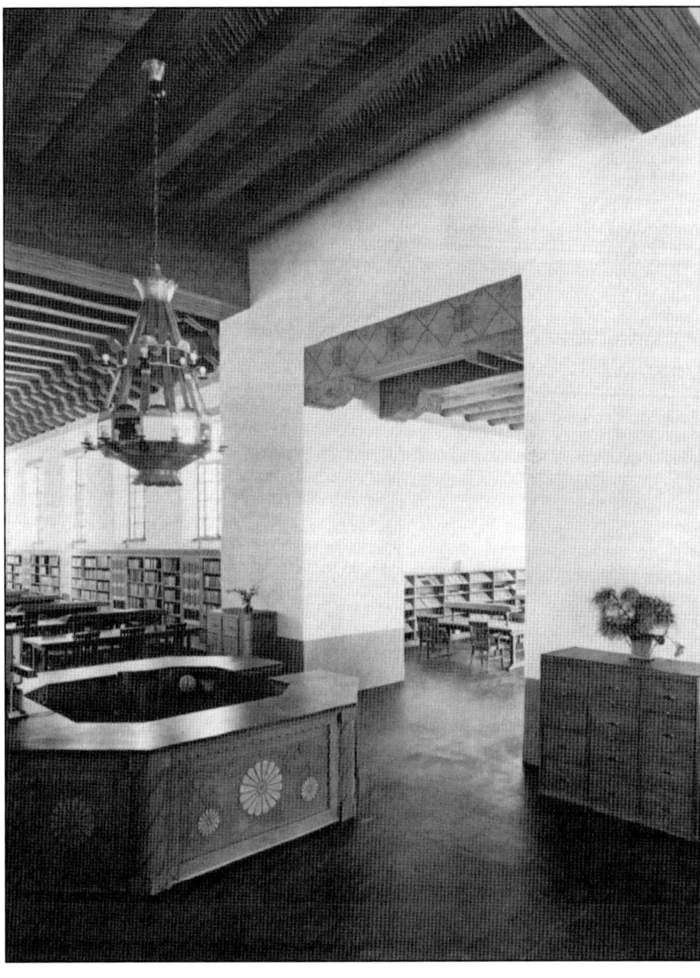

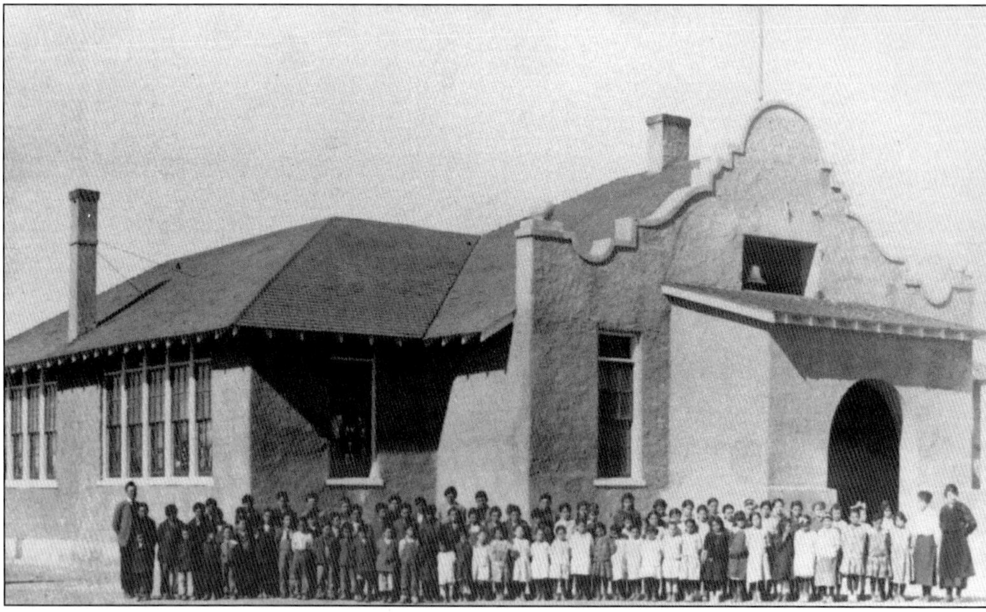

Los Padillas Elementary School as expanded in 1912 was located at the corner of Isleta and Los Padillas Road. At the time, it was called the most modern school in New Mexico. This not entirely successful rendering of the Mission Revival style look as though a bit of the Alvarado Hotel and the Isleta Convento were pasted onto a stucco box. With that said, it is typical of a number of public buildings from the time as Albuquerque explored regional architectural styling. (Courtesy of Nancy Tucker.)

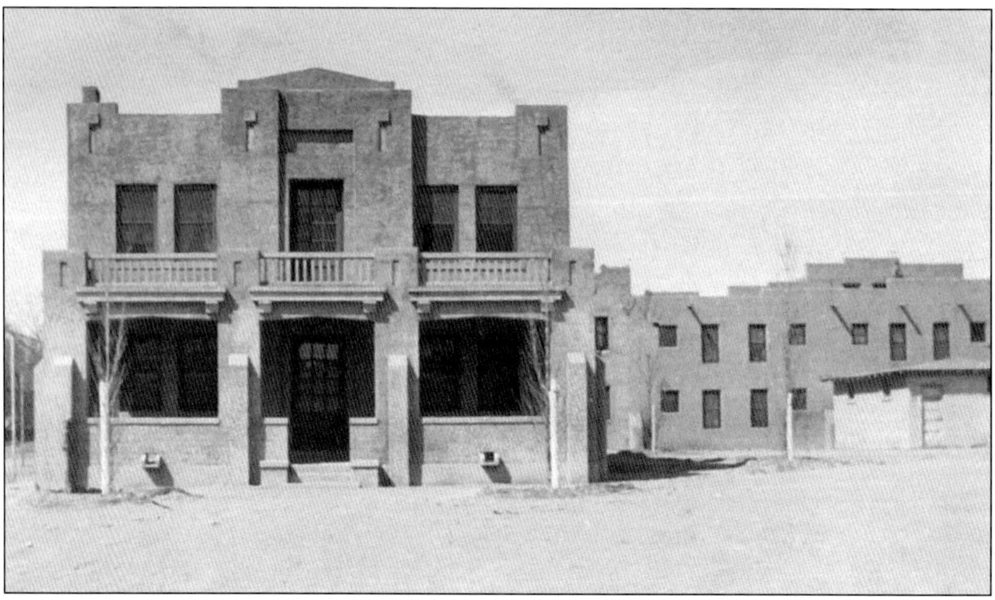

This now demolished UNM dormitory (1926–1927) comes from the awkward campus architectural period following George Tight and before John Gaw Meem. Stylistically, it is ambiguous and certainly not Spanish-Pueblo Revival or Mission. It has an almost Art Deco feel, especially if the second-level balcony railing were removed. (Courtesy of UNM CSWR Pauline Whitman Photograph Collection.)

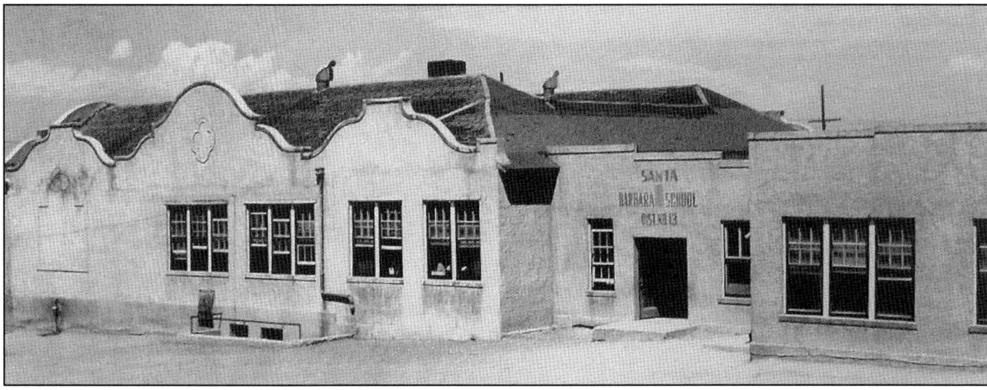

The Santa Barbara Elementary School, located in the Santa Barbara/Martineztown neighborhood, went through five major building phases between 1908 and 1938. Sometime after 1919, the present Mission-style parapet was added, resulting in a more successful "Alvarado Hotel" look than the earlier Los Padillas School effort. In 1992, it was renovated into eight apartments. (Courtesy of Nancy Tucker.)

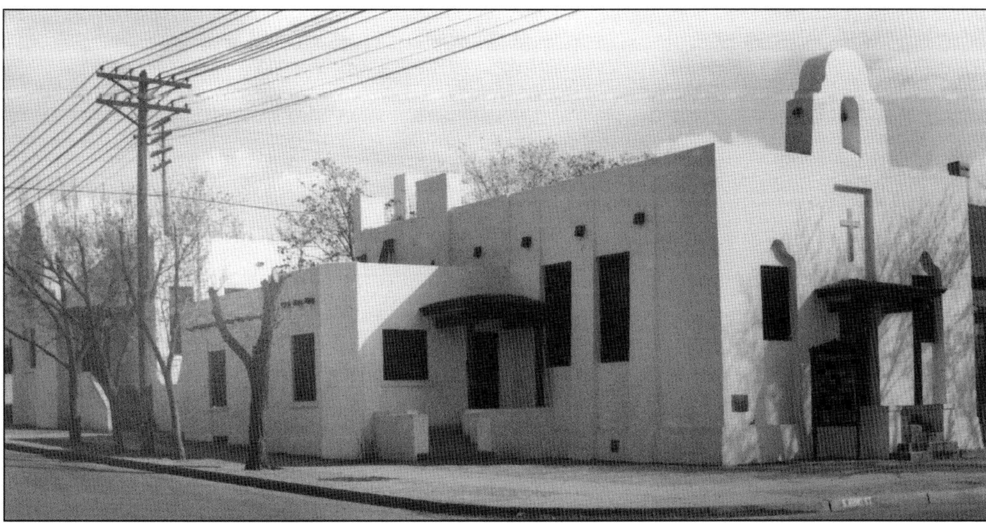

Pictured is the Immanuel Lutheran Church and School on South Arno Street around 1924. It has more of a Spanish-Pueblo feel than Mission Revival effect, despite its "mission" bell arch (see the Isleta Church, page 18). While the church and school are still active, apparently this building no longer exists. The form is stylized and modern, making for an interesting contrast to the UNM Chapel on page 24. (Courtesy of Nancy Tucker.)

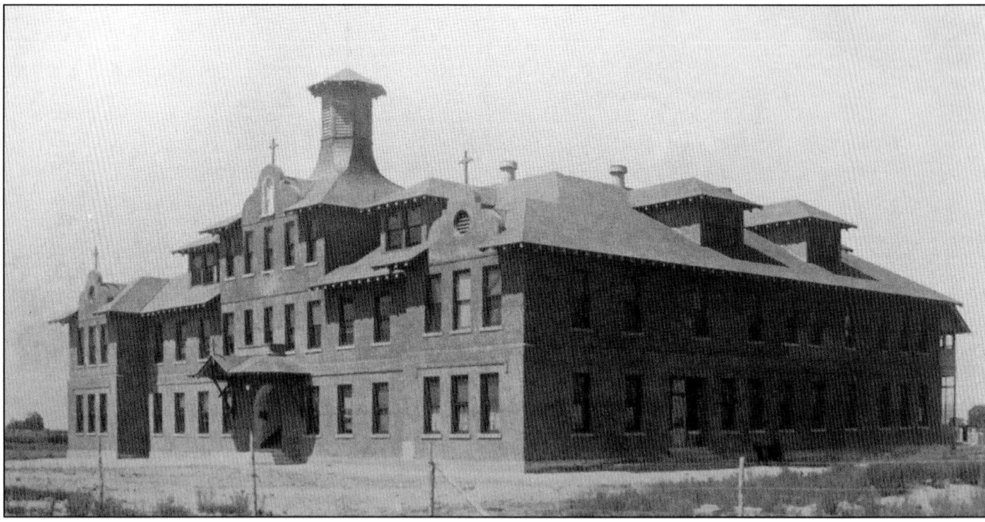

Just down the street from the Albuquerque Indian School (see page 32) on Indian School Road was St. Anthony's Orphanage and School. Founded in 1913 by the Sisters of the Order of St. Francis, it once housed as many as 400 boys. The original Mission-style building (above) was designed by Joseph L. LaDriere. The 1931 chapel addition (below) has a decidedly Roman Basilica quality. It was designed by self-trained Albuquerque architect Albert William Boehning (1891–1962). He helped establish the state's Architect Licensing Law and was New Mexico Registered Architect No. Four. (Above, courtesy of Nancy Tucker; below, courtesy of the National Archives, Historic American Building Survey.)

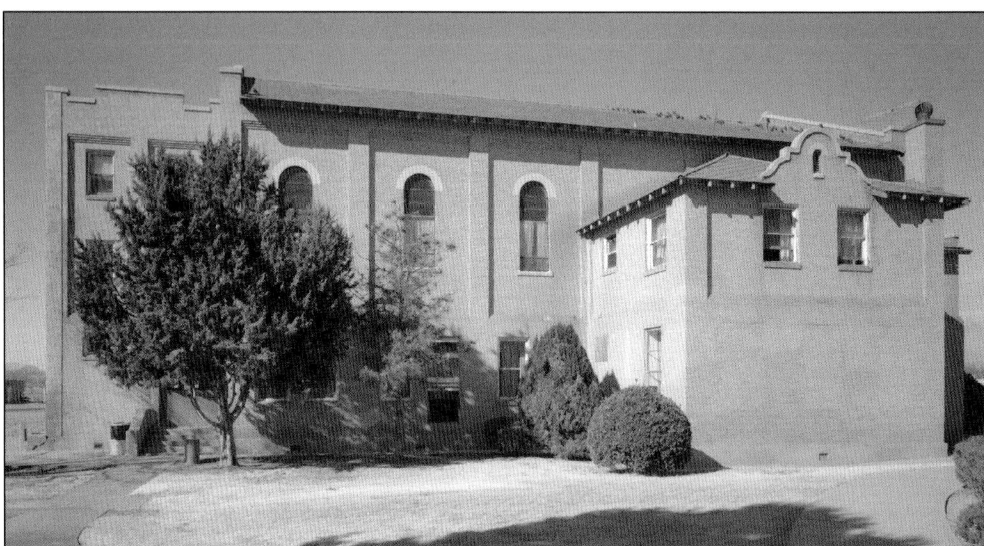

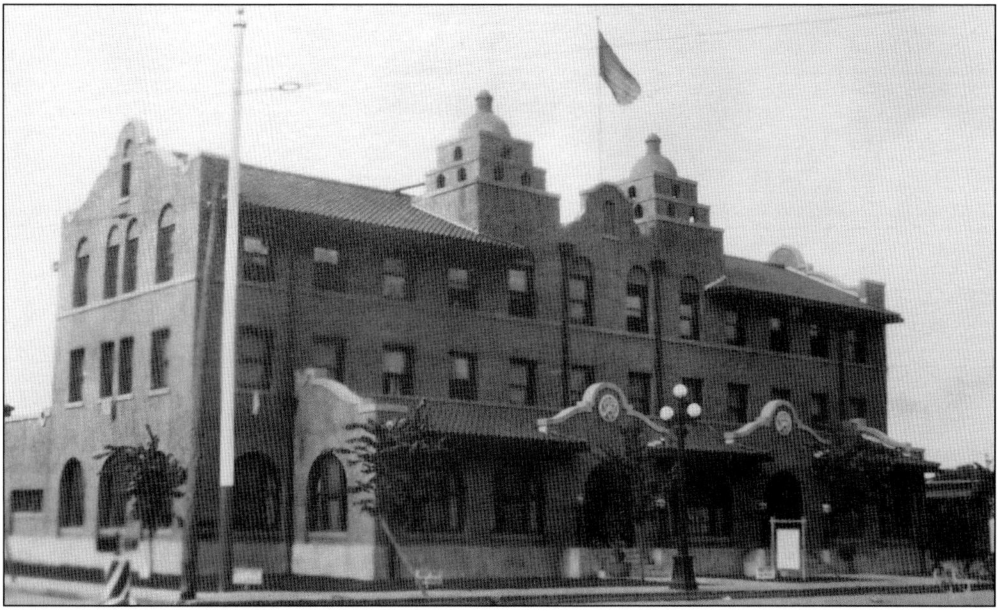

The Albuquerque YMCA was built in 1915 with community donations, which totaled $75,000. It was located on the corner of First Street and Central Avenue and just north of the Alvarado Hotel complex on land donated by the Santa Fe Railroad Company. This is a full-on Mission Revival building, designed to harmonize with the nearby Alvarado Hotel. (Courtesy of Nancy Tucker.)

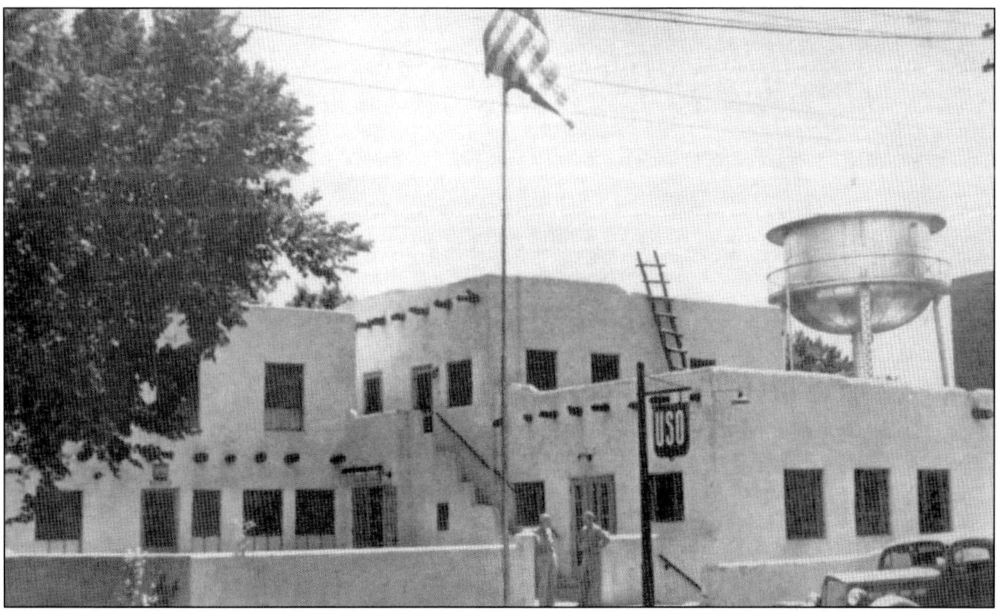

The USO opened in 1942 and closed in 1948 in a building that once served as the City Water Works at the corner of Broadway Boulevard and Tijares Avenue. That is a Packard parked in front; inside was a nickelodeon, bowling alley, and ping-pong table and on the radio, *Major Bowes Amateur Hour.* The building no longer exists. It is a typical 20th-century Albuquerque Pueblo Revival structure, possibly from the 1920s, complete with rustic roof ladder. (Courtesy of the City of Albuquerque, Historic Preservation.)

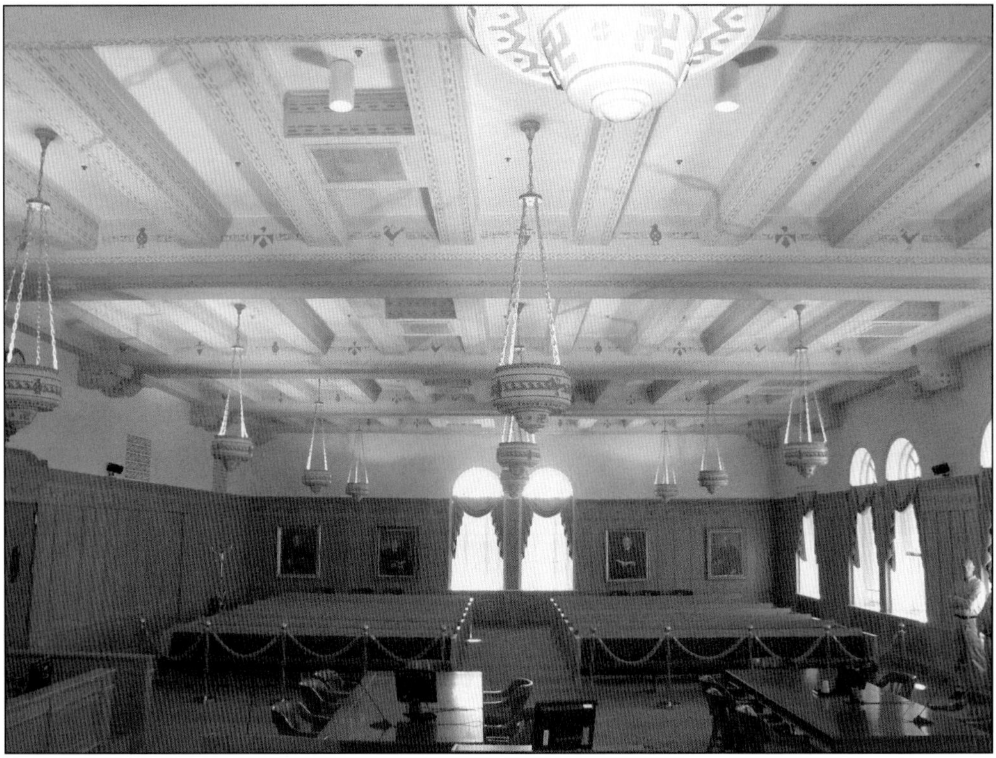

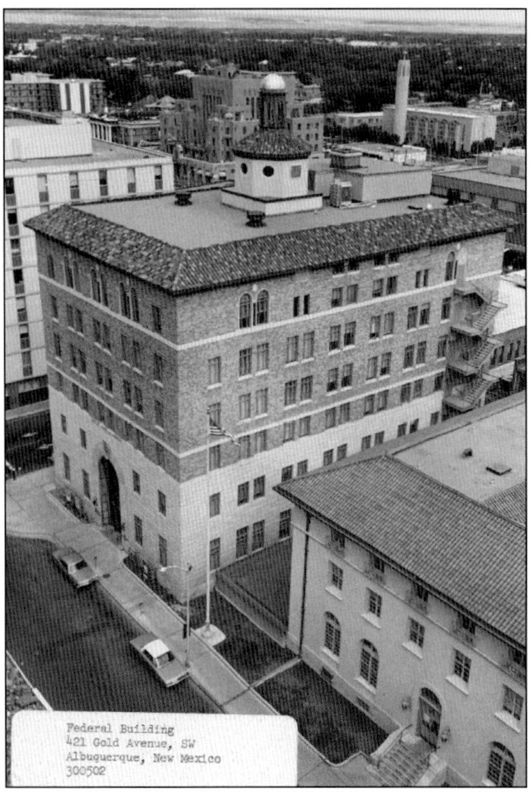

The federal courthouse, built in 1930 at the corner of Fifth Street and Gold Avenue, looks to be a typical Renaissance Revival Federal Building and is in harmony with the 1908 Mediterranean-style post office next door. However, the federal building is beautifully and extensively detailed with Native American southwestern motifs in terra-cotta reliefs and painted stenciled designs. Interior fixtures have a decidedly Art Deco feel. In addition, it contains several excellent WPA murals, including one of the 1680 Pueblo Revolt painted by Taos school artist Loren Mozley (1905–1989), a 1926 graduate of UNM. In 1982, the sixth floor courtroom was restored to its former glory. Once threatened with demolition, the building is a credit to the federal government and local preservation efforts. Today, the restoration looks like it was completed last week and not 30 years ago. (Both, courtesy of General Services Administration.)

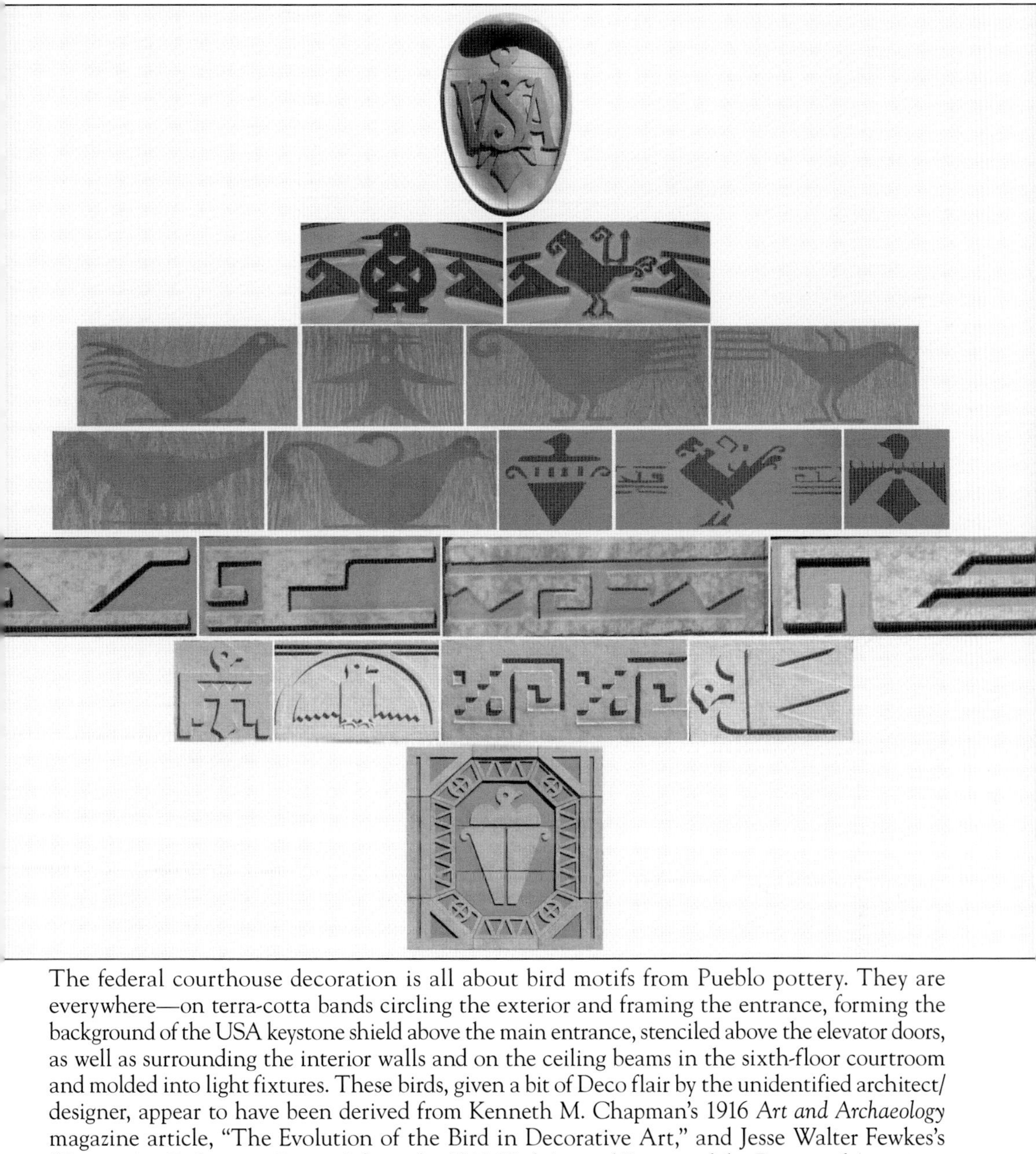

The federal courthouse decoration is all about bird motifs from Pueblo pottery. They are everywhere—on terra-cotta bands circling the exterior and framing the entrance, forming the background of the USA keystone shield above the main entrance, stenciled above the elevator doors, as well as surrounding the interior walls and on the ceiling beams in the sixth-floor courtroom and molded into light fixtures. These birds, given a bit of Deco flair by the unidentified architect/designer, appear to have been derived from Kenneth M. Chapman's 1916 *Art and Archaeology* magazine article, "The Evolution of the Bird in Decorative Art," and Jesse Walter Fewkes's "Designs on Prehistoric Pottery" from the 1919 33rd Annual Report of the Bureau of American Ethnology. (Courtesy of GSA.)

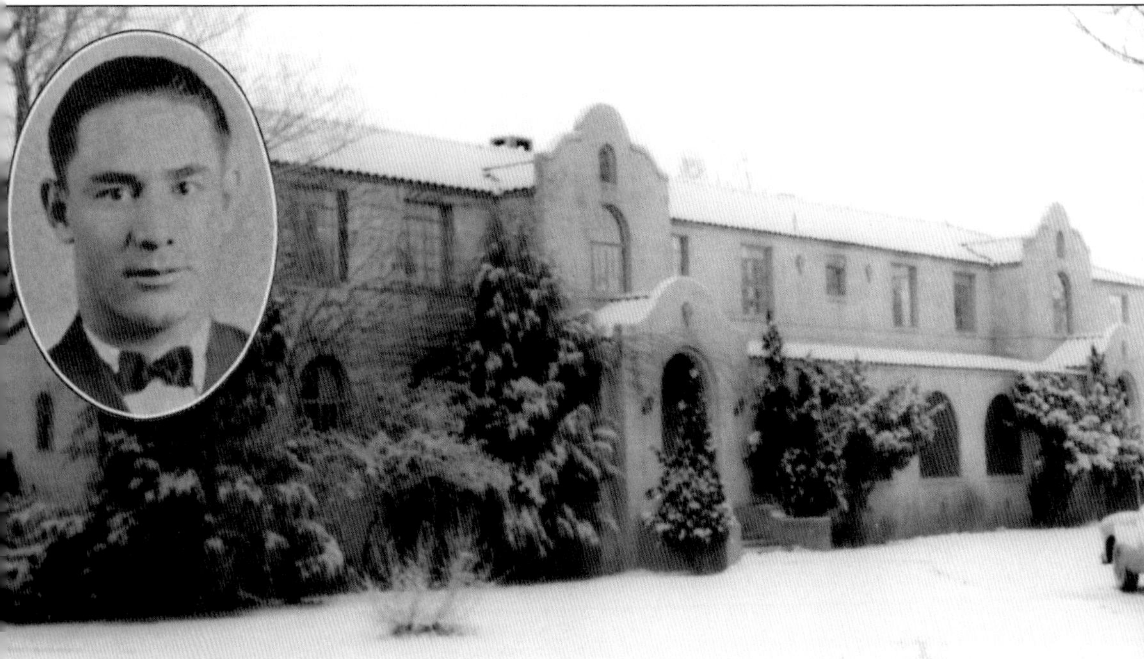

The Albuquerque Indian School (AIS) was established in 1881. By 1925, enrollment was over 800 students through the 12th grade. AIS continued operating until 1982. Sadly, the only remaining building is the 1931 Employee Dormitory and Club. It was designed and supervised by Joe Padilla, a recent AIS graduate, who was head of the school's carpentry department from many years. He was of Isleta and Hispanic descent. The use of a native architect is a singular achievement in Indian boarding school history as well as being apparently unique in Albuquerque. Student and faculty hands-on participation saved the government one-fourth of the total construction costs of $40,000. Note that the building is in the Mission Revival style; compare it with the Isleta Church on page 18. (Courtesy of Dr. Ted Jojola.)

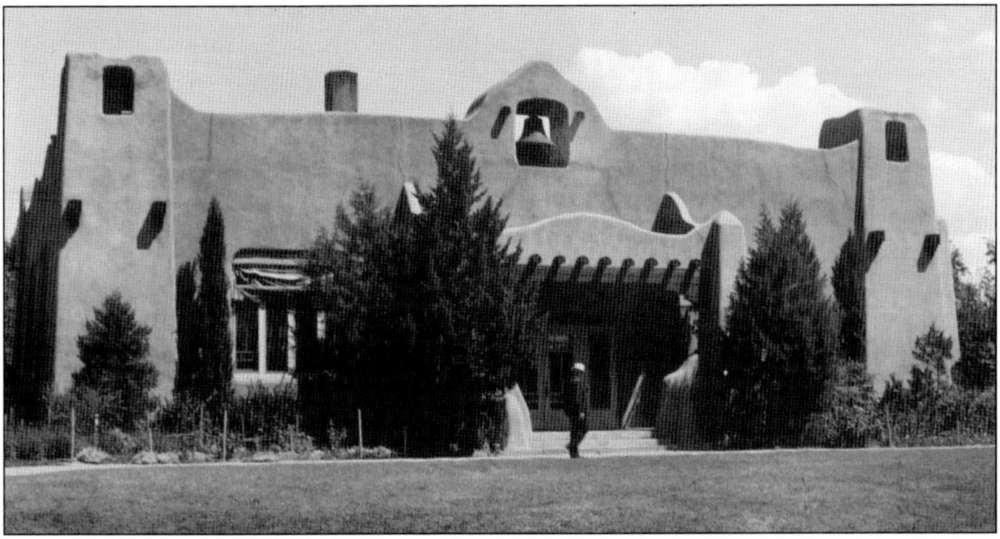

The Albuquerque Public Library, located at 433 Central Avenue, was designed by Arthur Rossiter and opened in September 1925. Restoration architect George Clayton Pearl states that the original construction "is the best example of its period and style in Albuquerque . . . rare in New Mexico . . . as most examples of the formative period . . . have been lost." Compare this structure's style to the Isleta Church on page 18. (Courtesy of Nancy Tucker.)

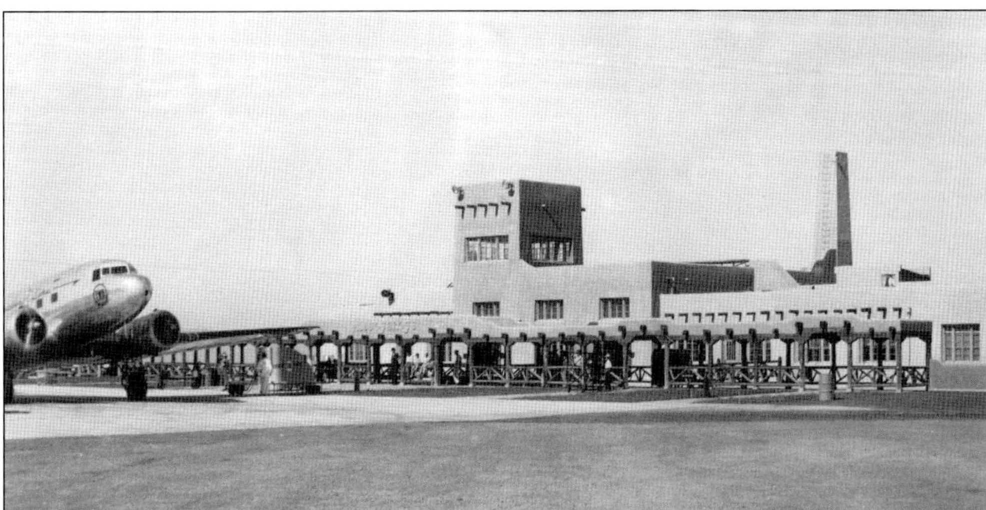

The 1939 adobe and steel Albuquerque Airport, a WPA project, is the city's first public air terminal. It was designed by city architect Ernest H. Blumenthal. The Pueblo Revival–style building's long covered colonnade with protruding roof *vigas* and rustic railing was a perfect staging area for arriving and departing passengers. (Courtesy of Nancy Tucker.)

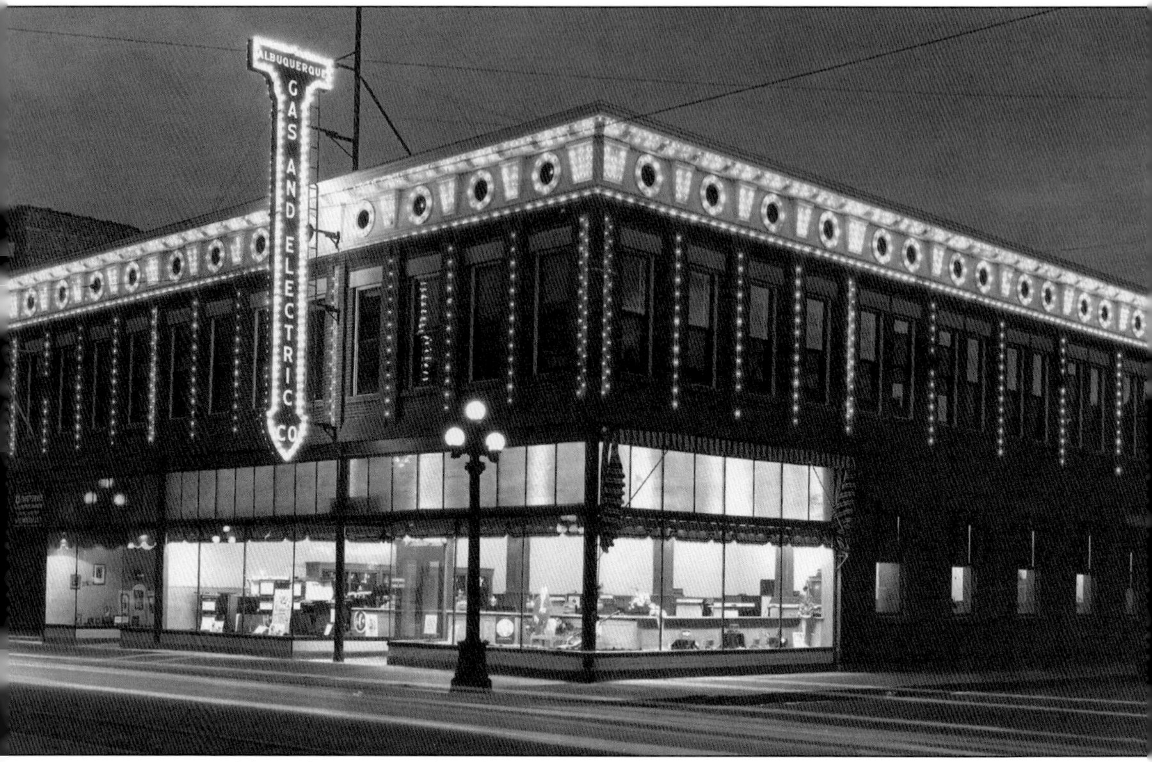

It is not Pueblo and not Deco, but the 1915 public service company building still stands at the southeast corner of Fifth Street and Central Avenue. Here it is in its full electric light show glory. Would that the original lighting scheme could be restored, perhaps with low power LEDs? What a wondrous complement to the Kimo Theater directly across the street. They both contrast dramatically with the styles of their respective decades—the Edwardian Era and the Roaring Twenties. (Courtesy of Albuquerque Museum.)

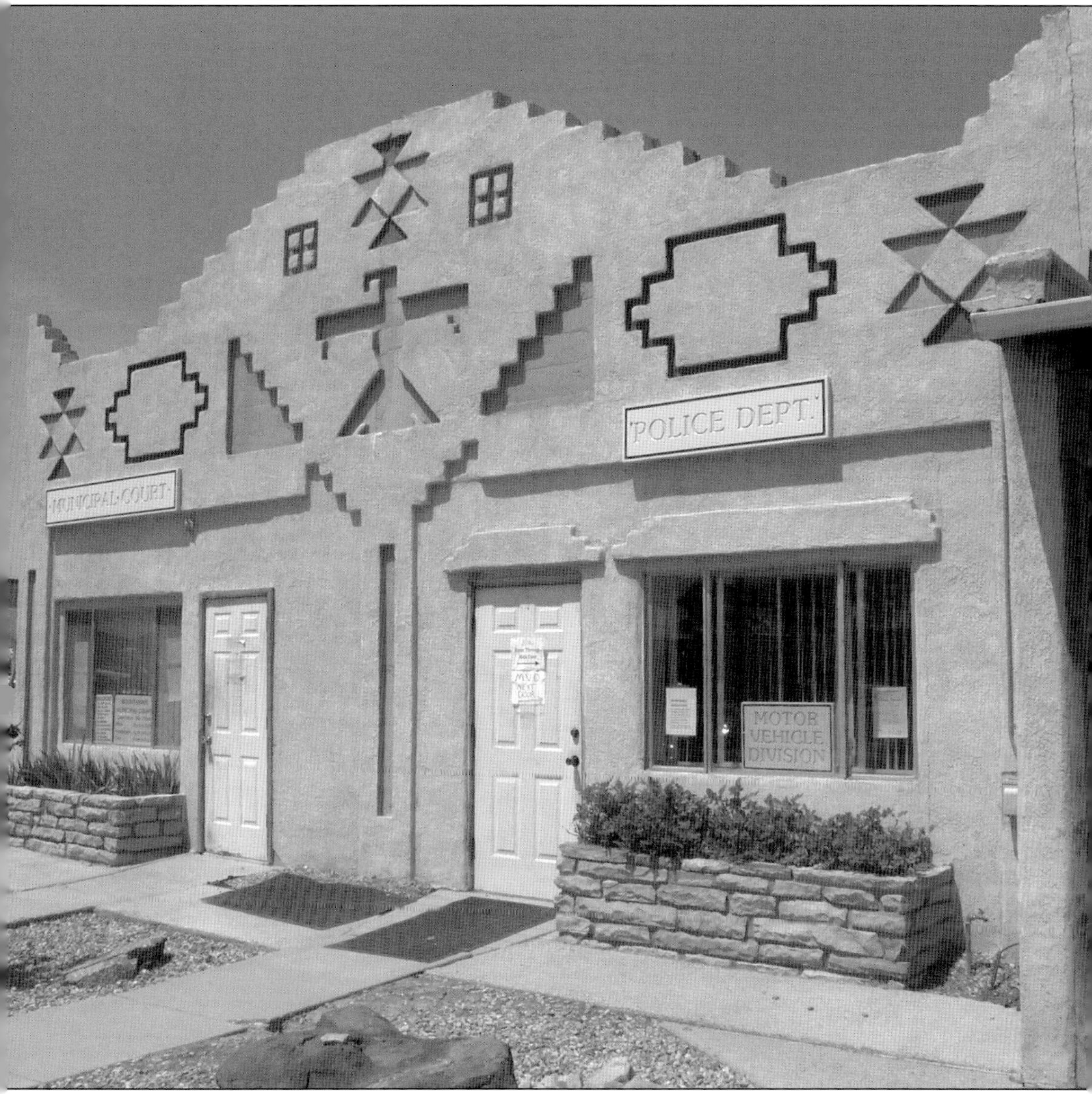

South of Albuquerque in Torrance County is the ranching and once farming town of Mountainair. It has some pretty interesting architecture, as seen later with the Shaffer Hotel. The Municipal Court and Police building was probably constructed in the mid-1920s. Complete with thunderbird and Indian designs, it might be called Vernacular Coyote Deco. (Author's collection.)

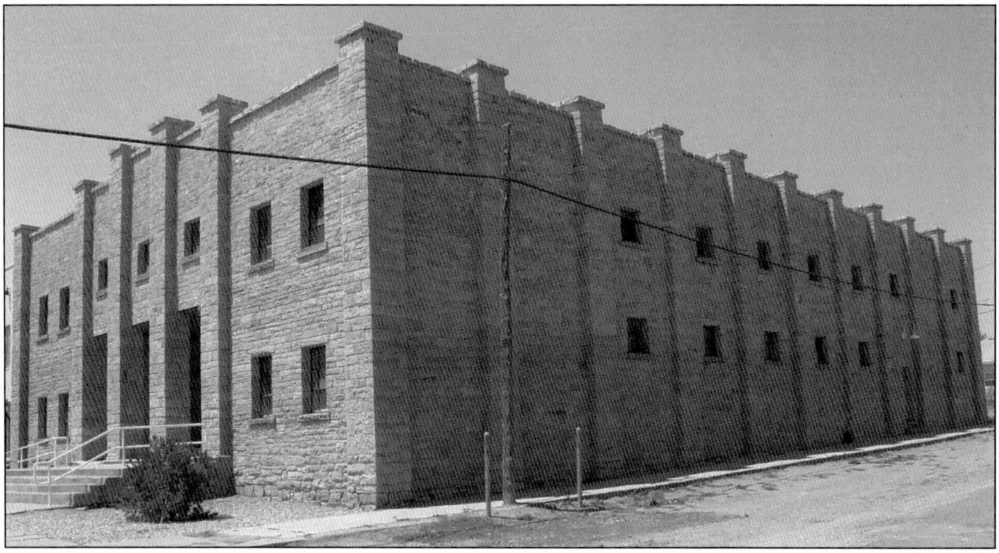

Here is the Mountainair mid-1930s WPA Community Center, now the Dr. Saul Recreation Center. It is a formal composition of local limestone and mortar, sans ornamentation, and is somewhat reminiscent of the massive Spanish church ruins at nearby Salinas Pueblo Missions National Monument. Like the building above, the Albuquerque Little Theater is essentially a big box. However, here is Territorial style (see the Hilton Hotel description on page 102), as interpreted by John Gaw Meem. This was a privately initiated WPA project; Harry L. Hopkins, national director and WPA director, as well as Lea Rowland, state WPA director, both attended the September 16, 1936, dedication. The mural by Dorothy Stewart, representing *Los Moros*, an early New Mexico folk play, was unfortunately destroyed by a 1961 remodel. (Author's collection.)

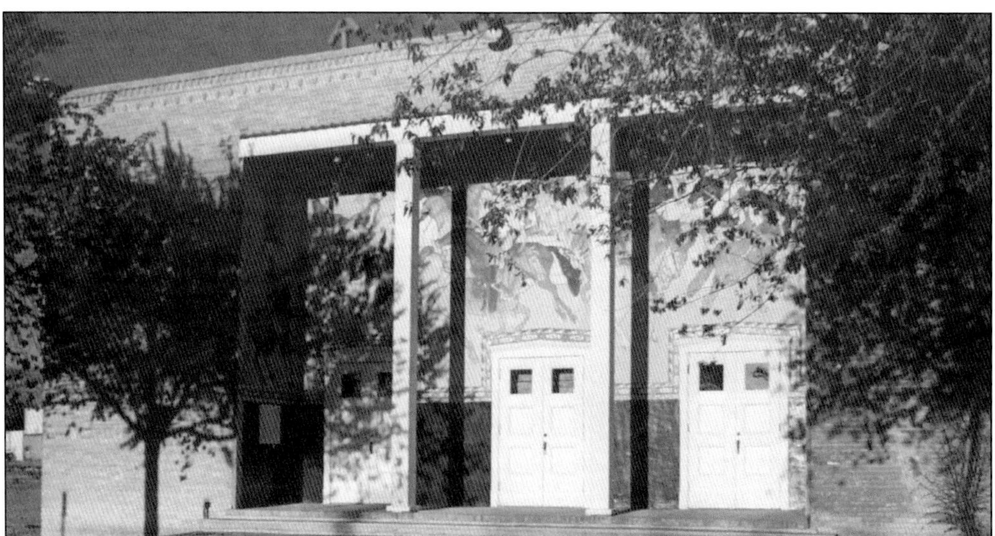

Three

Hospitals and Sanatoriums

Albuquerque was, and remains, the medical and health center of New Mexico. With its sunny weather and dry climate, it quickly drew health-seekers, especially those with tuberculosis. From the beginning of the 1900s through the 1930s, a sanatorium industry developed in New Mexico to serve the medical needs of patients suffering from tuberculosis, also known as consumption or the "White Plague." With railroad travel now within reach of the middle class, these sanatoriums were accessible to patients from across the country. A number of the sanatoriums were executed in the California-inspired Mission Revival style, and many were affiliated with religious organizations. The original Presbyterian Hospital complex is an important example of the early tuberculosis treatment centers. The Albuquerque Indian Hospital was first used as a sanatorium. Built near the University of New Mexico Medical Center in 1934 for the Department of the Interior, US Indian Service, Washington, DC, its National Register Nomination form states that "the Indian Hospital is the only building between Santa Fe and Socorro which combines the massing, vertical emphasis, materials, and detailing characteristic of [the] full-blown Art Deco style." A dramatic and colorful building, it is probably Albuquerque's best Art Deco building. Opening in 1932, the Albuquerque Veterans Affairs Medical Center (VAMC) blends Art Deco concepts with the Spanish-Pueblo Revival style. Contemporary newspaper articles state that the 15-building campus was planned to harmonize with the New Mexico scene and that the original main administrative building was modeled after the Taos Pueblo. The canteen and recreation building looks like a Spanish-period Pueblo church with Deco-inspired corner towers. Smaller residential buildings are essentially Pueblo Revival–style bungalows. In addition to Pueblo and Spanish influences, there are Mayan arches as well as idiosyncratic Art Deco details. The VAMC has grown into a massive complex of buildings, but fortunately the earliest structures have been preserved.

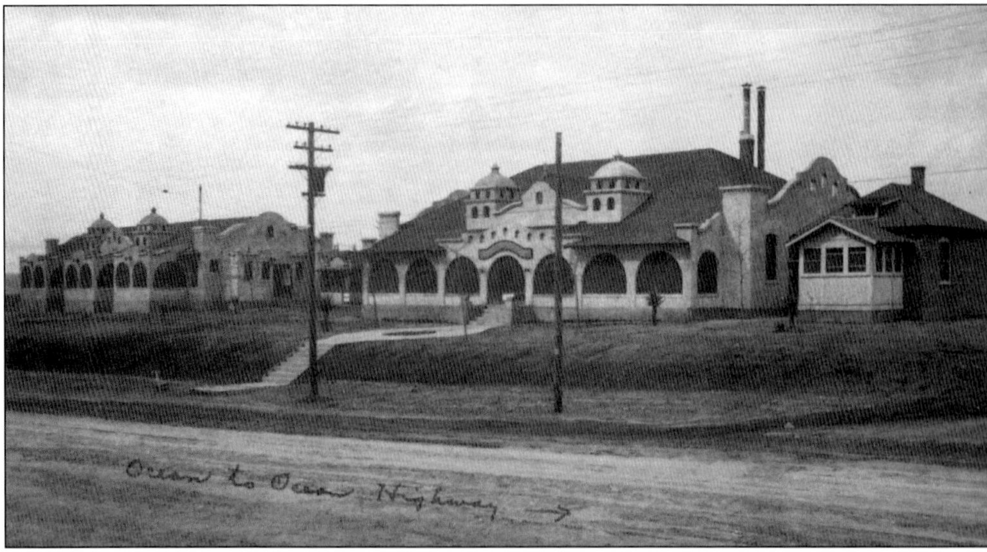

The Methodist Women's Home Missionary Society operated hospitals countrywide. Their Albuquerque Methodist Deaconess Sanitarium opened in 1912 with 66 beds. These c. 1916 structures in Mission Revival style were on Central Avenue west of UNM and were most likely modeled after California types. However, they echo New Mexico forms (see the Isleta Church on page 18), while the towers are similar to what was originally found on several New Mexico churches. (Courtesy of Nancy Tucker.)

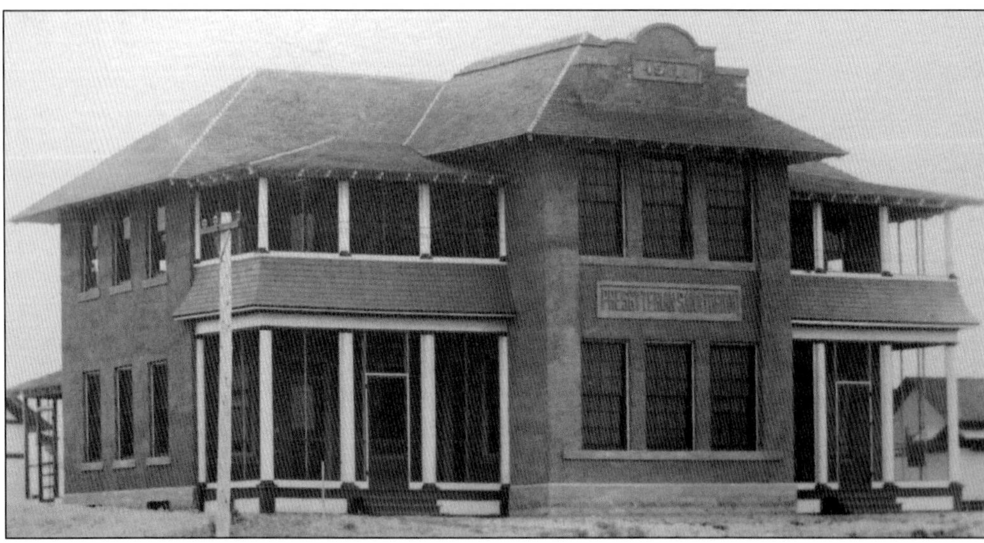

This 1911 building, with a slight nod to the Mission Revival style, is the first significant structure of the Presbyterian Sanatorium, originally organized in 1908. It initially served tuberculosis patients. By 1918, it had become a large complex, as it is today. The 1931 Maytag Research Center, one of E.B. Cristy's last designs, is the only surviving early building, a two-story box with a Mannerist and Renaissance entrance. (Courtesy of Nancy Tucker.)

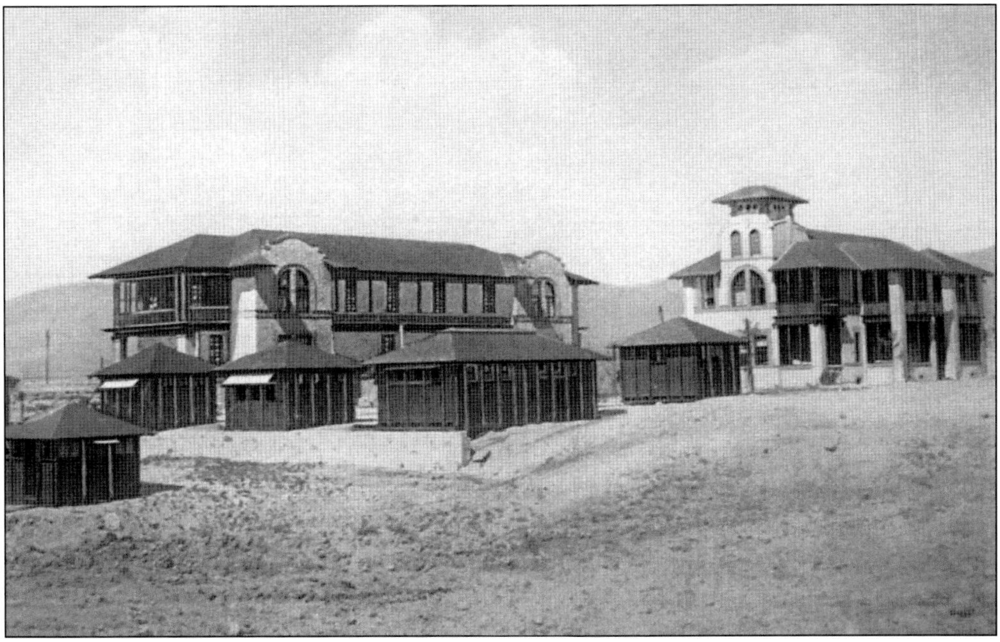

Dr. Abraham Given Shortle (1871–1922) was the first tuberculosis specialist in Albuquerque and in 1908 founded the city's first sanatorium, seen here. These buildings also allude to the Mission Revival and have interesting split arch windows. Shortle was an important figure in the early development of the city, active in both city and state affairs. The Shortle Sanatorium became the Albuquerque Sanatorium, and Shortle was later director of St. Joseph's Sanatorium. The picture below is identified as the annex to the National Lutheran Sanatorium. This is clearly a later, early 1920s, view of one of Shortle's original buildings. The Albuquerque Sanatoriums have a complex history, going through a number of ownerships and ultimately coalescing into some of the city's major medical institutions. (Both, courtesy of Nancy Tucker.)

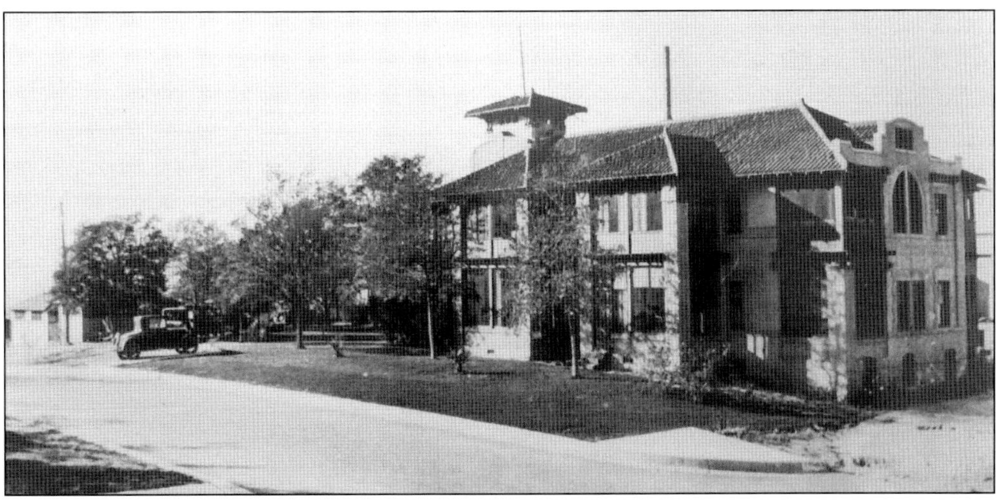

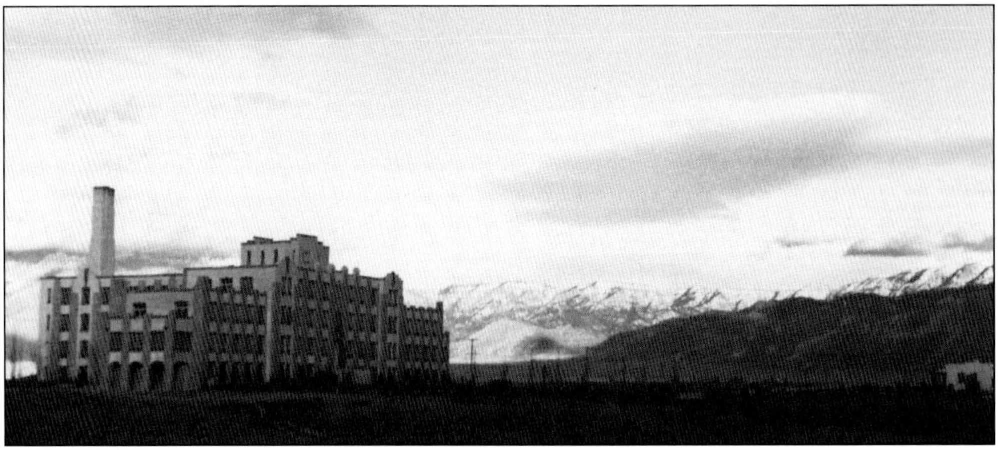

These pictures show the 1934 Albuquerque Indian Hospital, originally a tuberculosis hospital, before encroaching development spoiled its dramatic setting and a front entry addition completed in 1982 spoiled its front elevation. Fortunately, the building remains mostly intact. Pictured below are the original formal steps leading to the pronounced entry of the main lobby. While evoking Pueblo forms, such as the stepped pilaster tops, the structure contrasts dramatically with the Pueblo Revival buildings on the nearby UNM campus. Peach and turquoise terra-cotta bands and details highlight architectural forms. The hospital still serves the Native American community, and in this case primarily the Navajo. The building, as a whole, reflects well on a new attitude toward Native America health care that began with the presidency of Franklin Roosevelt. (Both, courtesy of Nancy Tucker.)

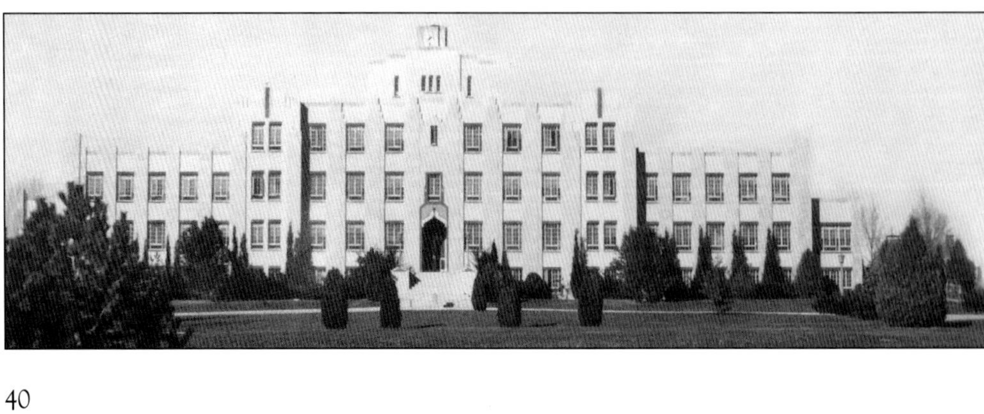

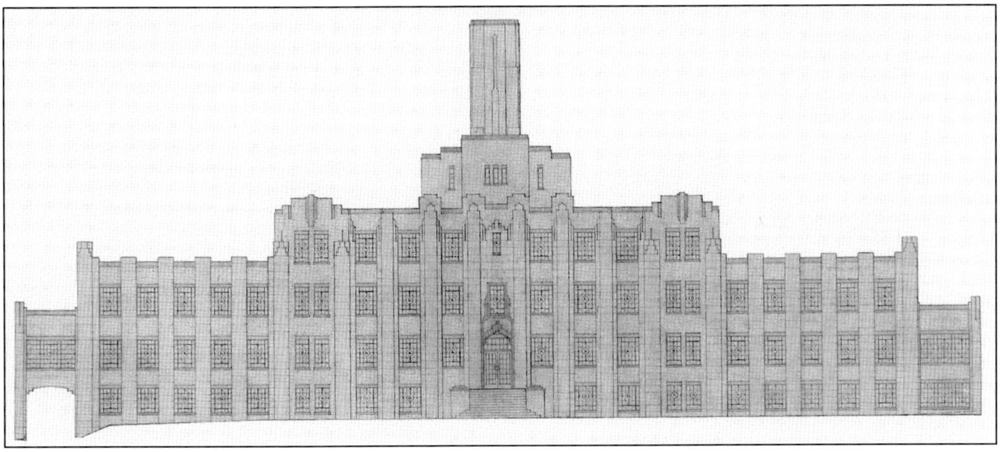

Albuquerque Indian Hospital was the first Bureau of Indian Affairs (BIA) building not constructed to a standard design. Chief BIA architect, Hans R. Stamm (1884–1966), who lived in Washington, DC, was instructed to take regional architectural features and motifs into consideration. Clearly, he most successfully absorbed a southwestern aesthetic. The south elevation is pictured above and the north elevation below. The vertical nature of the design is evident, making the building seem much larger from a distance. This well proportioned and elegant structure, at the peak of modernity for its time, has a strong regional feel. (Both, courtesy of the UNM CSWR, Sanatorium, and Hospital Plan Collection.)

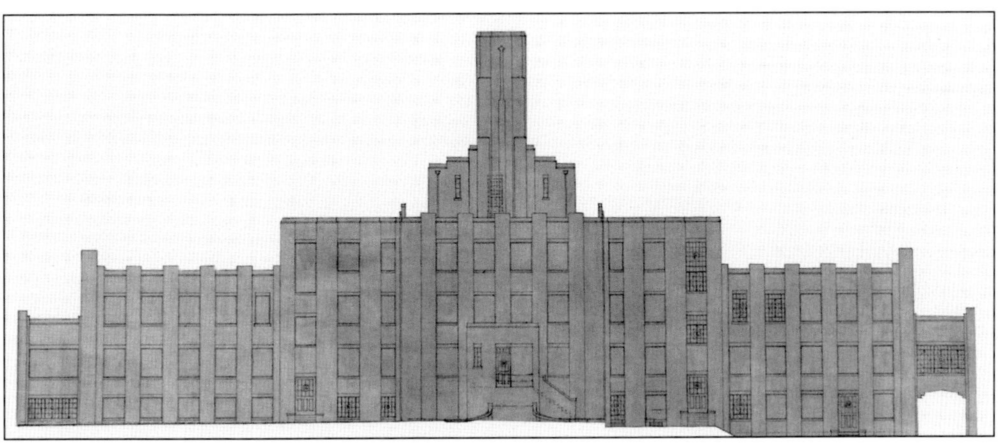

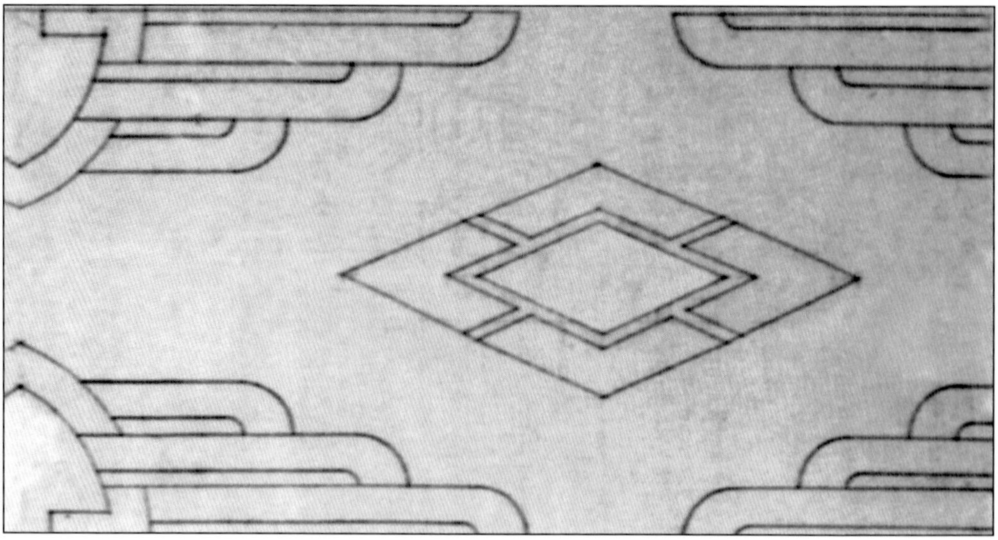

Stencil detailing and pilasters with designs derived from Navajo rugs survive in the lobby of the Albuquerque Indian Hospital. Pictured here are some renderings of original stencil designs. They are identifiable to particular rug types that became formalized during the 1920s. Bands, diamonds, and pyramid shapes decorate the walls and ceiling in red, blue, green, and mustard yellow. In addition, there is a Navajo man's profile, a specific reference to the hospital's primary users, in the center of the lobby's linoleum-tiled floor. (Both, courtesy of the UNM CSWR, Sanatorium, and Hospital Plan Collection.)

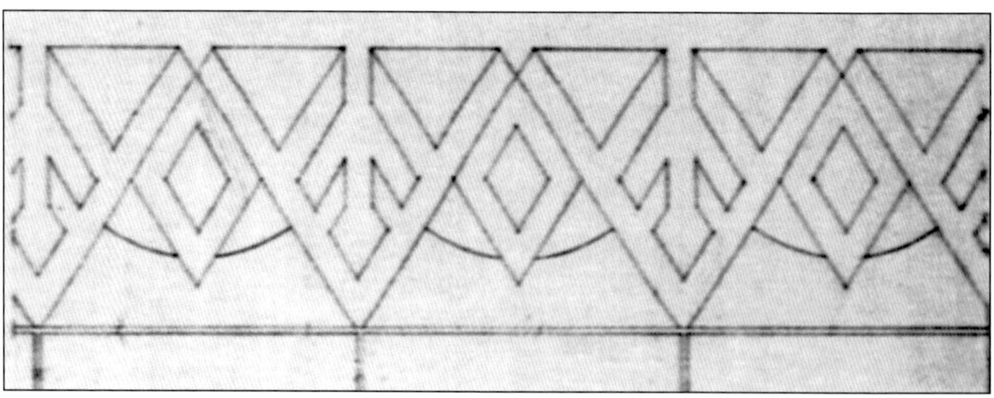

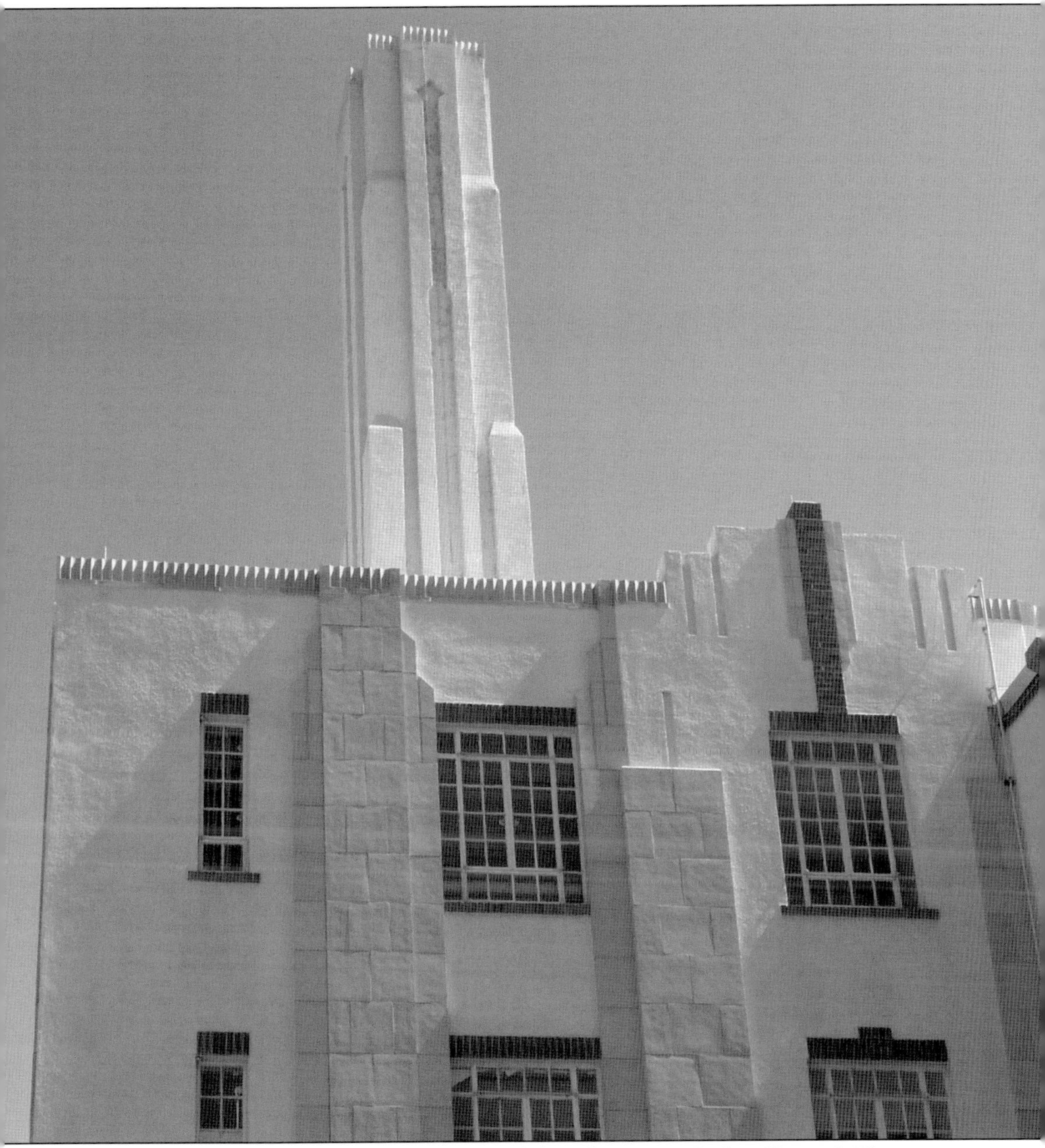

This image shows detail of the eastern elevation of the Albuquerque Indian Hospital. The tower with the incised arrow is the incinerator smoke stack. Fluted cornice pieces of turquoise-colored terra-cotta edge the parapet, contrasting with the yellow terra-cotta of the pilasters and the redbrick window detailing. "Cloud-lift" and stepped motifs are also clearly visible. Native American influences are paramount, yet the execution is pure Art Deco. (Courtesy of US Department of Health and Human Services.)

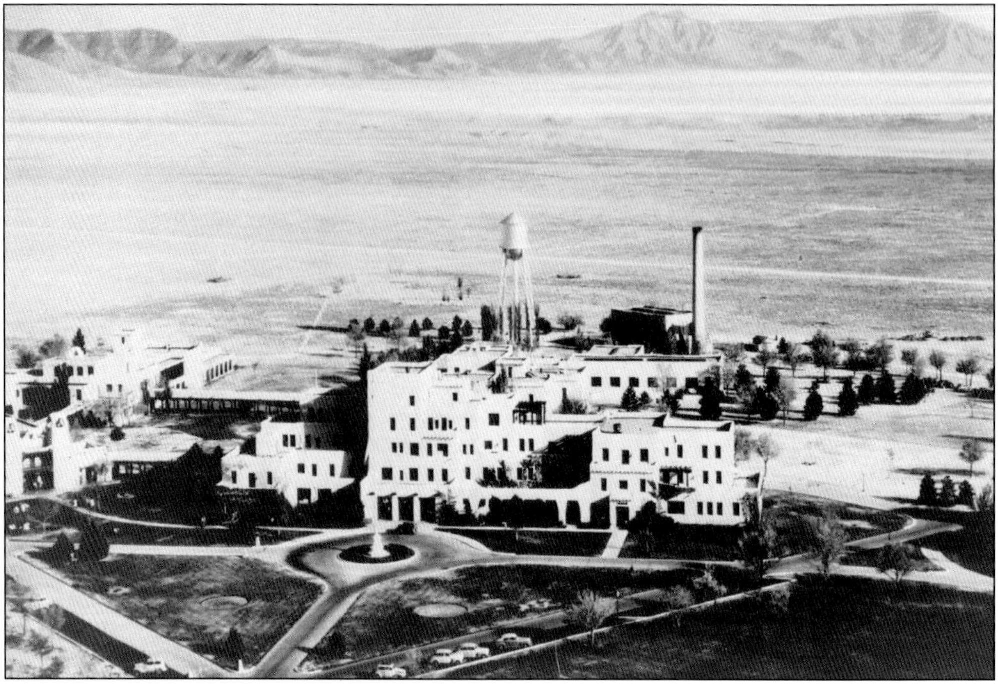

The Albuquerque Veterans Affairs Medical Center (VAMC) admitted its first patient in 1932. The 516-acre complex with 15 buildings originally housed 262 patients and cost $1,125,000. As with the previously discussed Albuquerque Indian Hospital, an effort was made to develop a design scheme that reflected the New Mexico region. However, in this case, the architects from Washington, DC, decided to adhere more strictly to the Pueblo Revival style. Even so, this was the 1930s, and Art Deco and Spanish architectural forms crept in. The overall plan does a fine job of connecting the various buildings with covered walkways, some with upper and lower decks. While overall building forms are in keeping with Spanish-Pueblo Revival massing, it seems that several architects were involved with the design of specific structures. (Both, courtesy of the National Archives, Historic American Building Survey.)

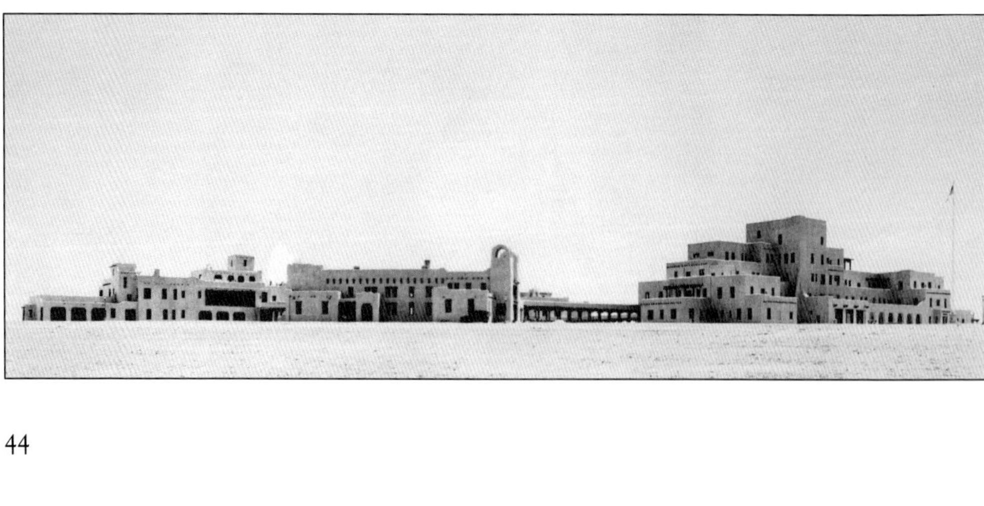

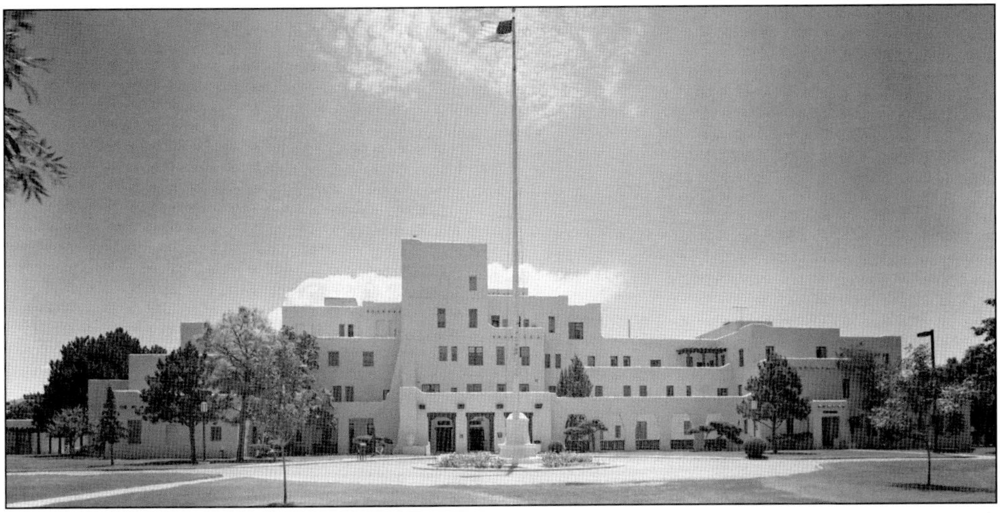

The above photograph is of the VAMC's main administration building as originally constructed and as it appears essentially unchanged to this day. Below is a US Historic American Building Survey (HABS) elevation of a portion of the northern house block of Taos Pueblo. Although it is continually renewed, the building form at this site may be at least 1,000 years old. The influence of Taos Pueblo on the hospital building is unmistakable. There is a clear correspondence in overall building massing and in details, such as the large protruding *vigas* (ceiling beams.) A striking difference, which blends remarkably well with the overall design of the building, is a large front patio framed by Mayan arches. These arches are seen again at the Franciscan Hotel (pages 98–101), which predates the building by 12 years. (Both, courtesy of the National Archives, Historic American Building Survey.)

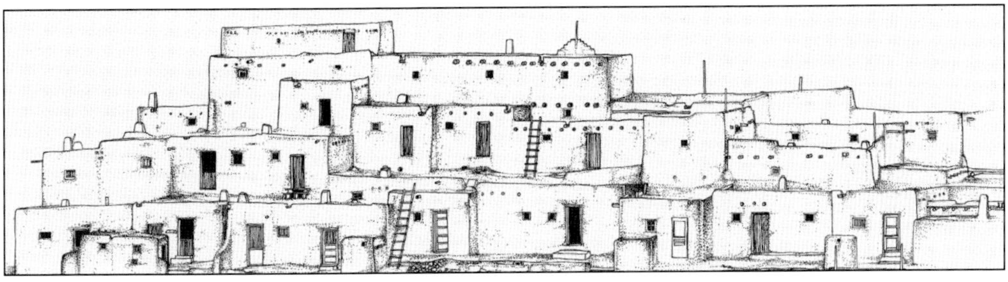

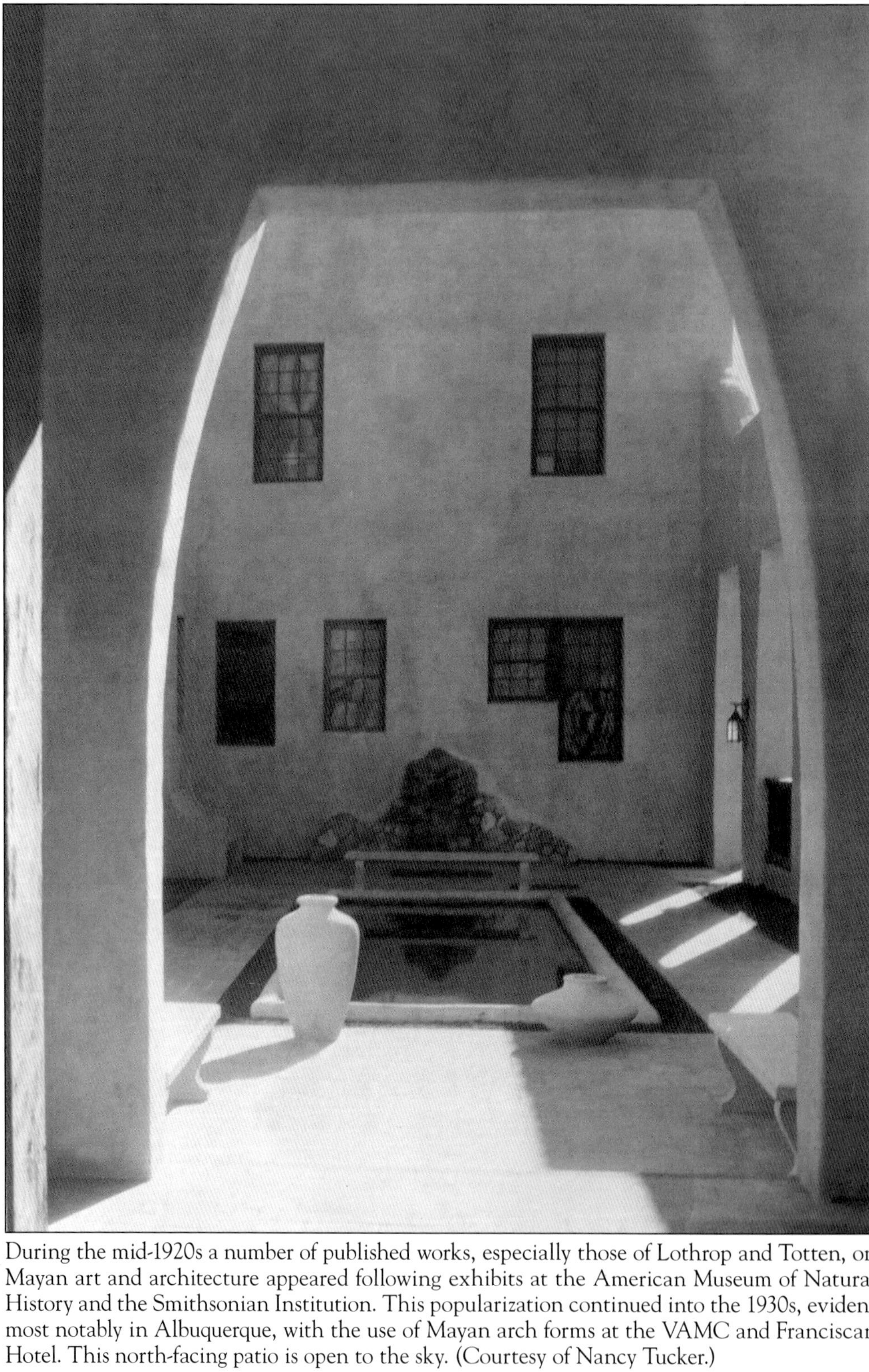

During the mid-1920s a number of published works, especially those of Lothrop and Totten, on Mayan art and architecture appeared following exhibits at the American Museum of Natural History and the Smithsonian Institution. This popularization continued into the 1930s, evident most notably in Albuquerque, with the use of Mayan arch forms at the VAMC and Franciscan Hotel. This north-facing patio is open to the sky. (Courtesy of Nancy Tucker.)

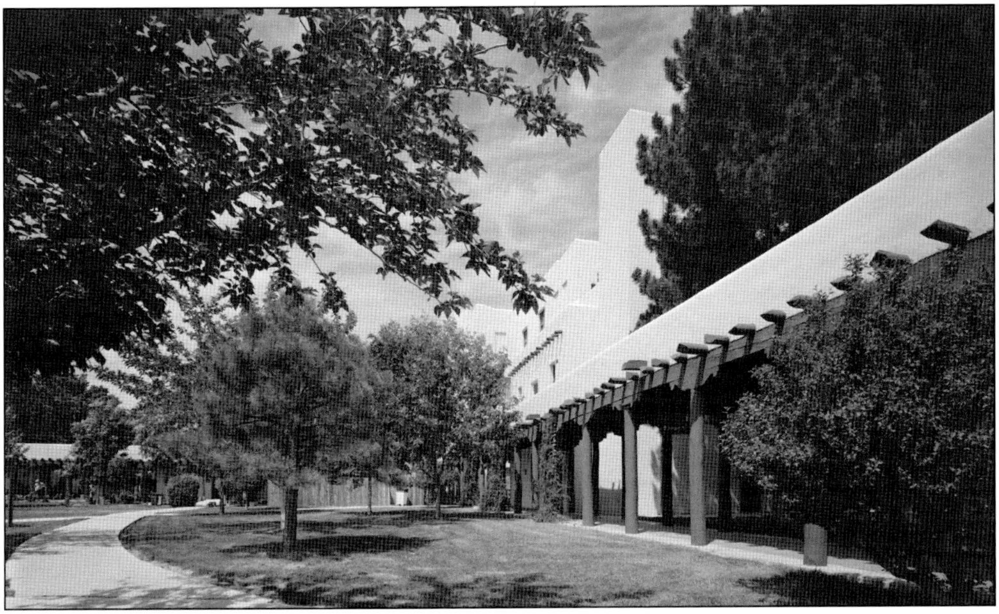

Patios and walkways are an integral part of the VAMC plan. At the top, there is a Pueblo Revival–covered and ramada-like walkway connection to the main building with dining and recreation facilities. The photograph below is another view of the courtyard patio, fronting the main building. The Mayan arch colonnade framing the Sandia Mountains is especially picturesque. (Both, courtesy of Nancy Tucker.)

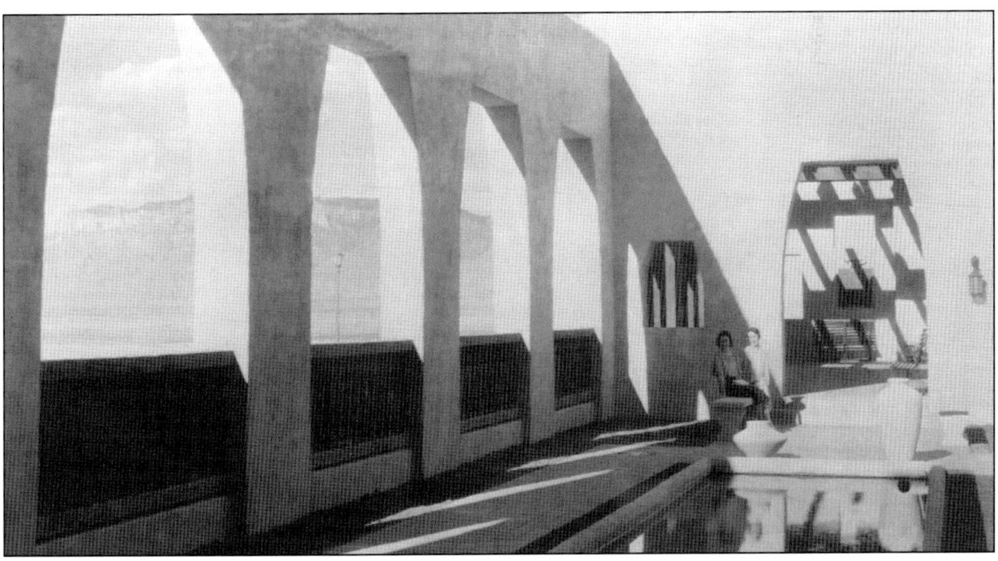

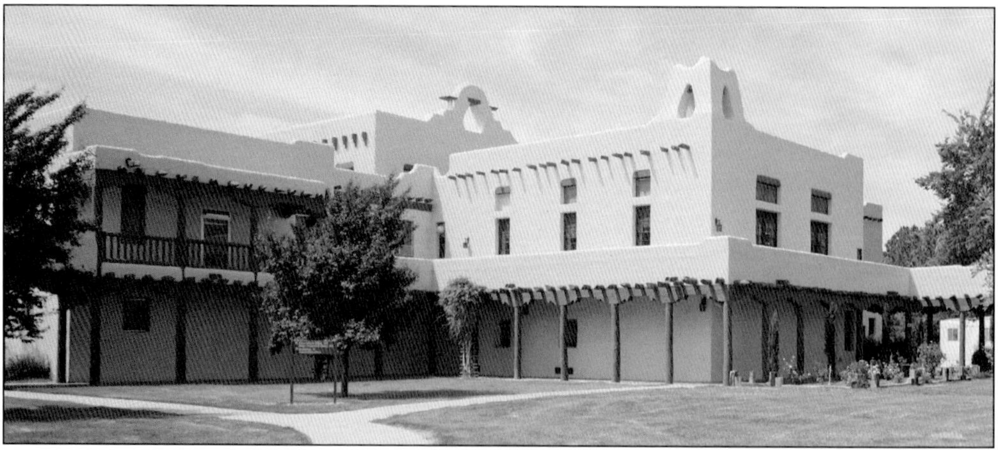

The Spanish church tower of the VAMC Canteen and Recreation Building, pictured on page 13, is mirrored in the Art Deco corner tower of the original Pulmonary Care Building, pictured above. Note the rather odd placement of a bell arch on another building behind it. Once again, there are covered colonnades, walkways, and a second-floor covered porch. (Both, courtesy of the National Archives, Historic American Building Survey.)

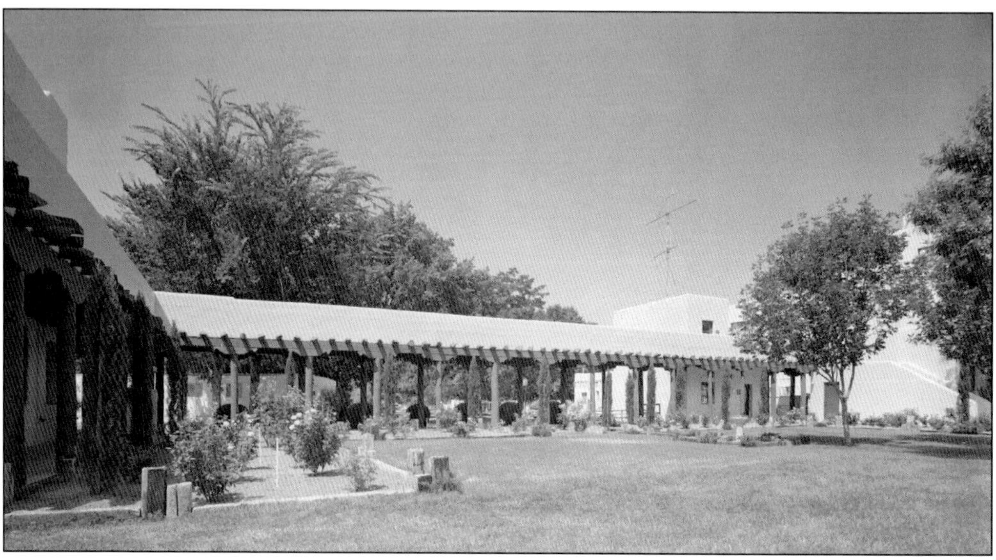

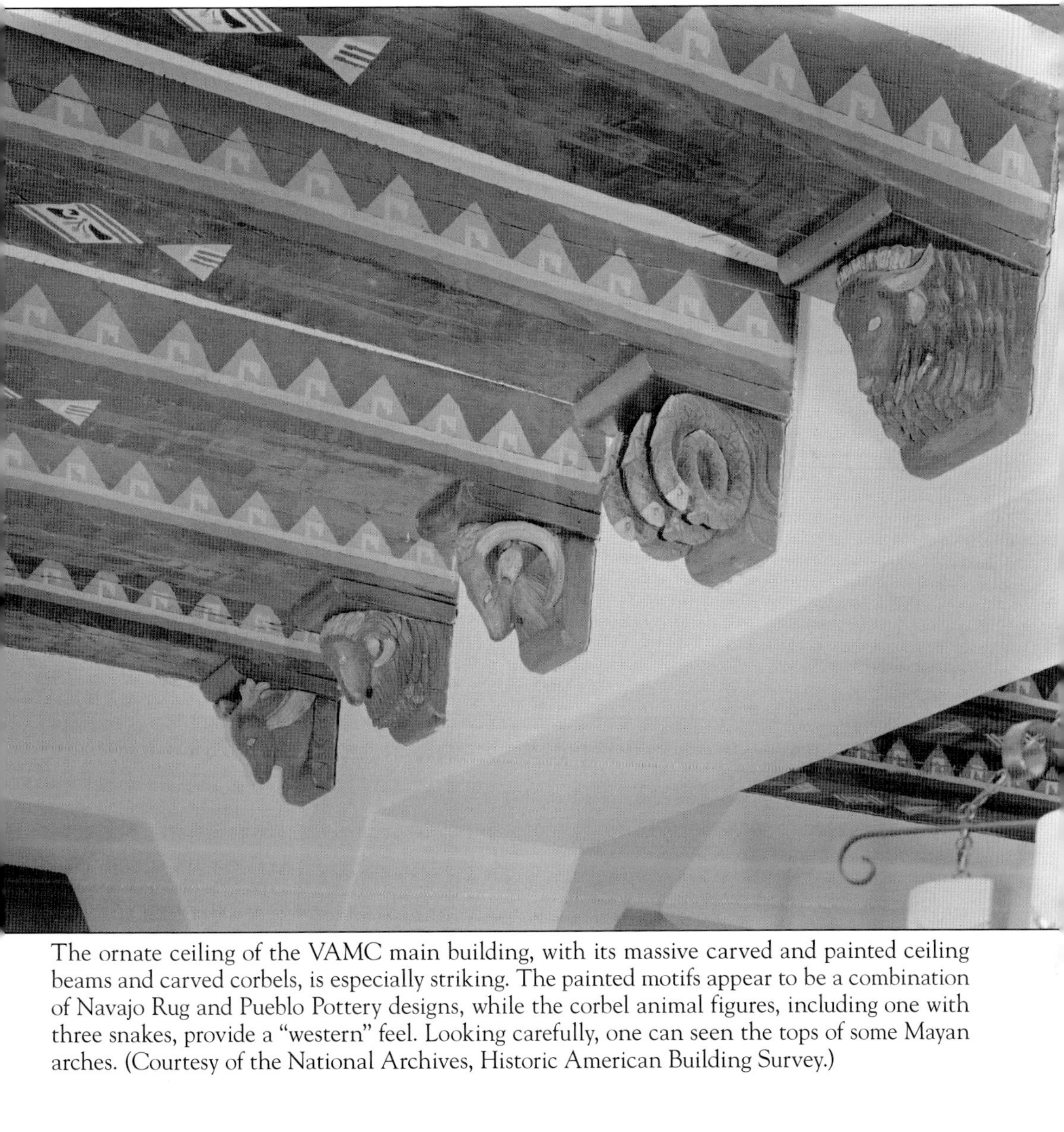

The ornate ceiling of the VAMC main building, with its massive carved and painted ceiling beams and carved corbels, is especially striking. The painted motifs appear to be a combination of Navajo Rug and Pueblo Pottery designs, while the corbel animal figures, including one with three snakes, provide a "western" feel. Looking carefully, one can seen the tops of some Mayan arches. (Courtesy of the National Archives, Historic American Building Survey.)

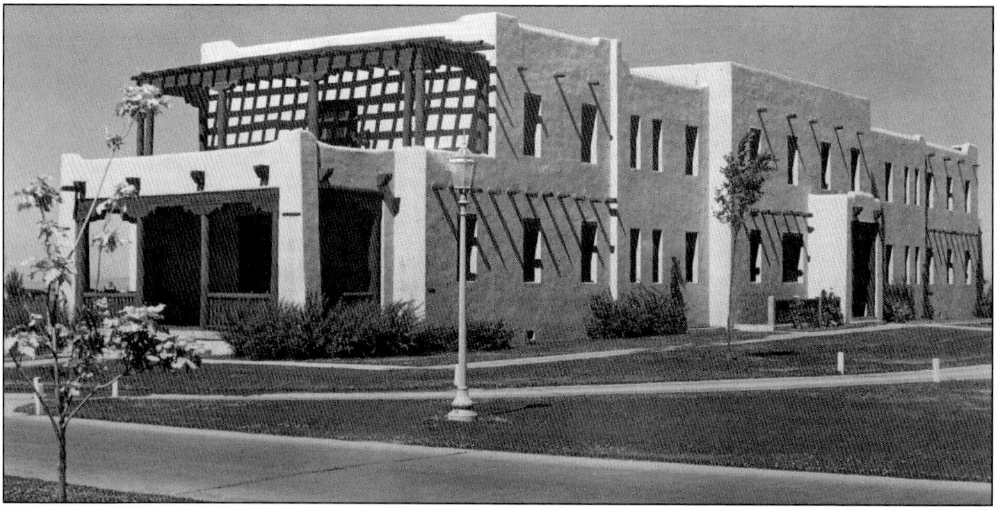

The hospital complex includes a number of residential buildings and clinics. Above is the original nurses home. The structure below also originally served as a staff quarters. Essentially, all of these smaller buildings are in a strict Pueblo Revival style with covered porches. (Both, courtesy of the National Archives, Historic American Building Survey.)

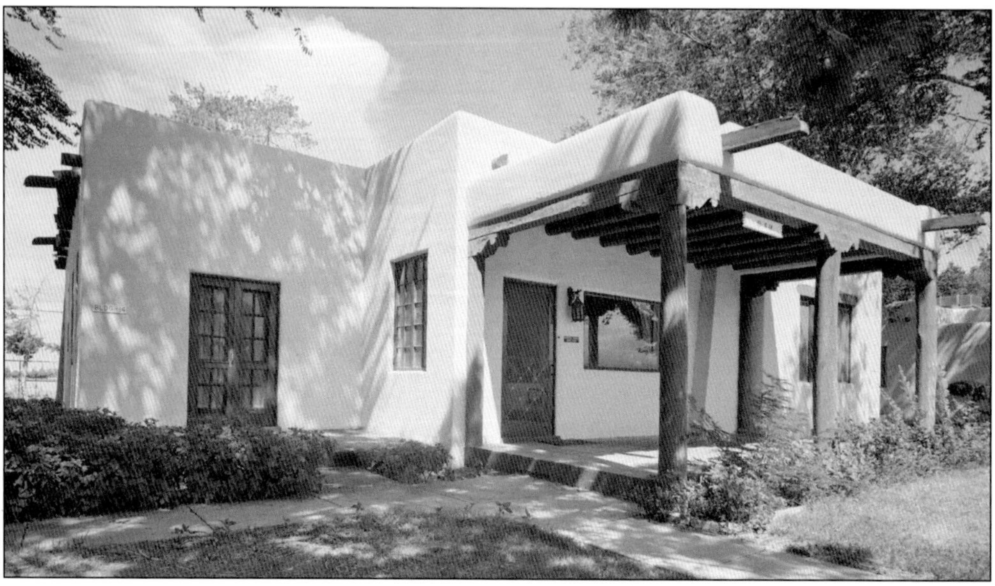

Four

Commercial Buildings

It is with the architecture of Albuquerque's commercial buildings that the full flowering of this book's themes play out. While the architecture of Santa Fe ossified into its vision of a mythic past, Albuquerque's development was, for all intents and purposes, unrestrained. The up and coming movers and shakers were free to express their view of the modern and attract as much attention to their commercial enterprises as they could. The striking southwestern landscapes and rich cultural mixing profoundly influenced the city's architecture. Native American influences, a key focus of the book, are realized to their fullest in the pseudo pueblo of Wright's Trading Post, the lavish interior of the Kimo Theater, and the striking blend of traditional and modern of Maisel's storefront. Strong "pure" Art Deco designs, in both its 1920s and 1930s iterations, are well represented in the city's downtown commercial buildings. The Court Café, the Skinner Building, and Fremont Grocery are especially good examples of Art Deco retail buildings found throughout the county at the time. There are also some eclectic buildings in Albuquerque that did not entirely fit with this book's themes; however, they just could not be left out. These include a life insurance company in a Venetian Doges Palace, an Egyptian wool-warehouse, and a Mayan industrial building. Also included are a couple of buildings that were never constructed. One is on the business promotional piece that opens this chapter, and the other is a wonderful Art Deco skyscraper by John Gaw Meem that, when it finally was built in the 1960s, had become a clichéd glass box of the time. With a few exceptions, Route 66 gas stations and cafés have been excluded since they are well presented in a number of books on Route 66, such as Arcadia Publishing's *Route 66 in New Mexico.*

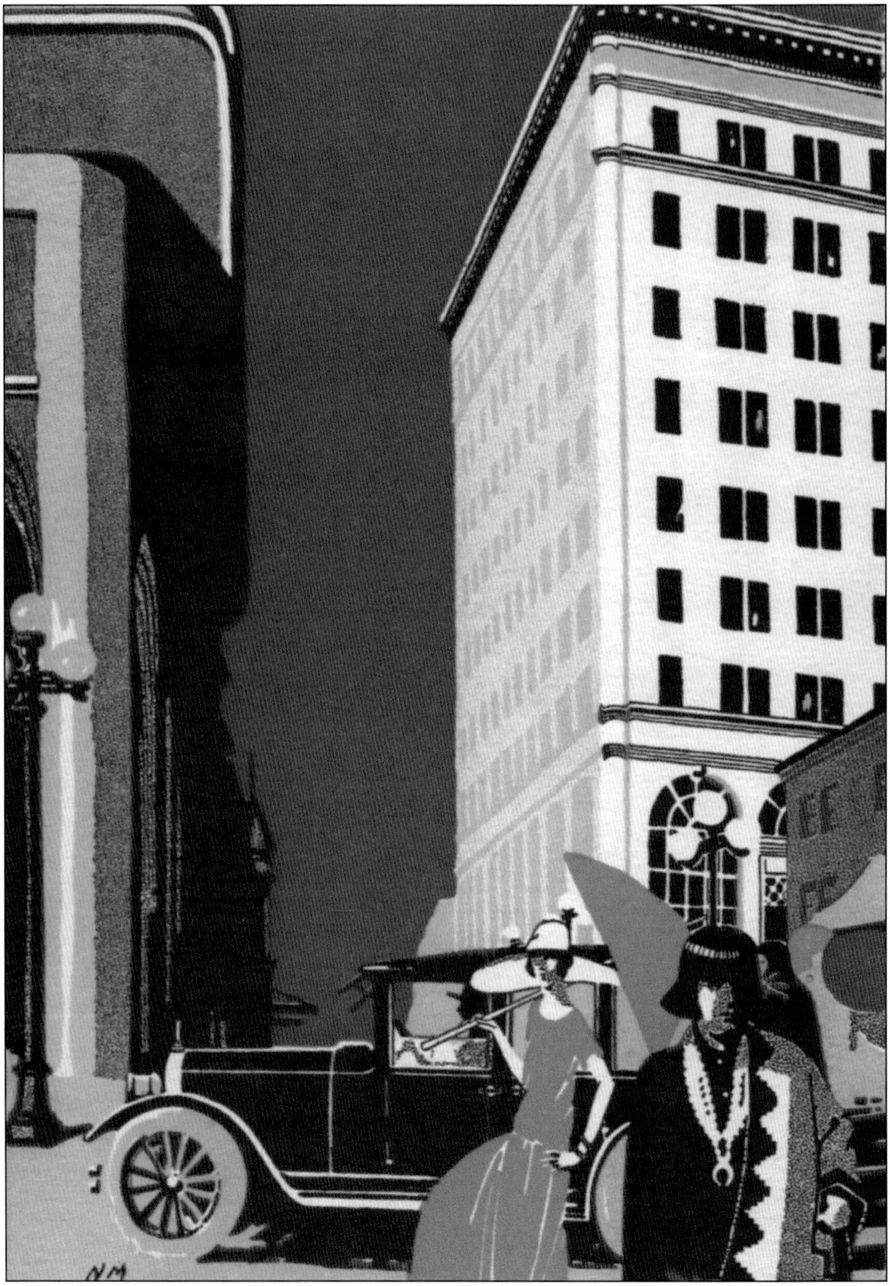

This illustration is from a business promotional brochure, "Forty-two Years of Banking Service in New Mexico," which was put out in 1925 by the First National Bank of Albuquerque. The scene is of the north corner of Central Avenue and Third Street. The building on the right is the 1922 First National Bank, designed by Trost & Trost, important regional architects of the time working out of El Paso, Texas. The building to the left with the curved cornice is entirely an invention of the artist Hazel Gruehl, who was with the Howard Gruehl Advertising Agency. The car and fashionably dressed young woman show a modern age, and the Native American with blanket and silver necklace lets one know he or she is in the Southwest. (Courtesy of the UNM CSWR Brochure and Flyer Collection.)

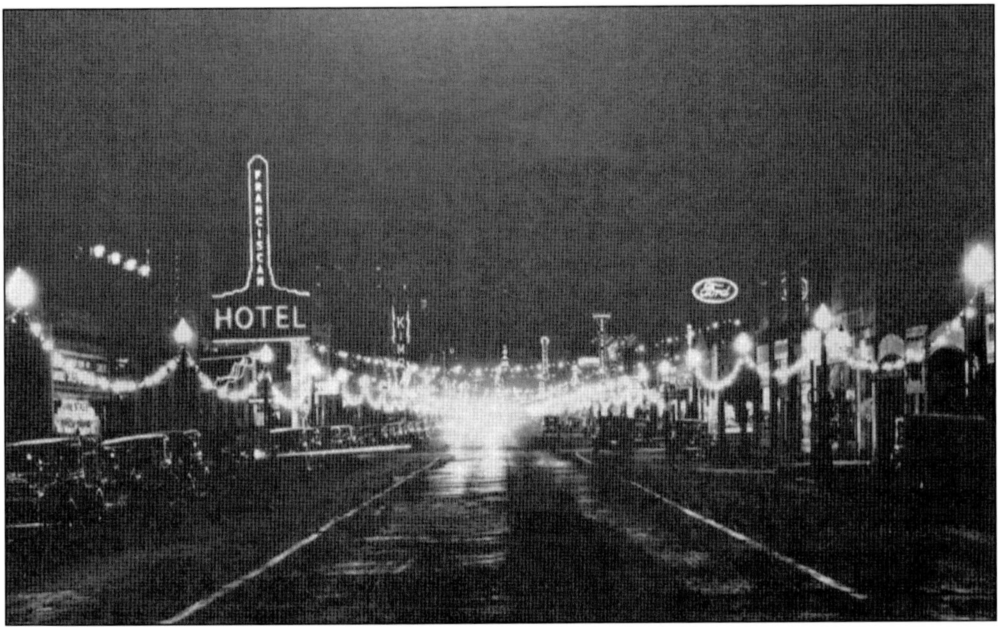

Many buildings in this chapter front on a six-block length of Central Avenue called downtown Albuquerque or "New Town," which distinguishes it from the pre-railroad "Old Town." The next six images are a drive down Central Avenue from west to east, or roughly from Sixth Street to Fourth Street. Looking down Central Avenue from Sixth Street is the dominant Franciscan Hotel, and in mid-block is the Kimo Theater. The tall building at the end of the street on the left is the First National Bank. (Both, courtesy of Nancy Tucker.)

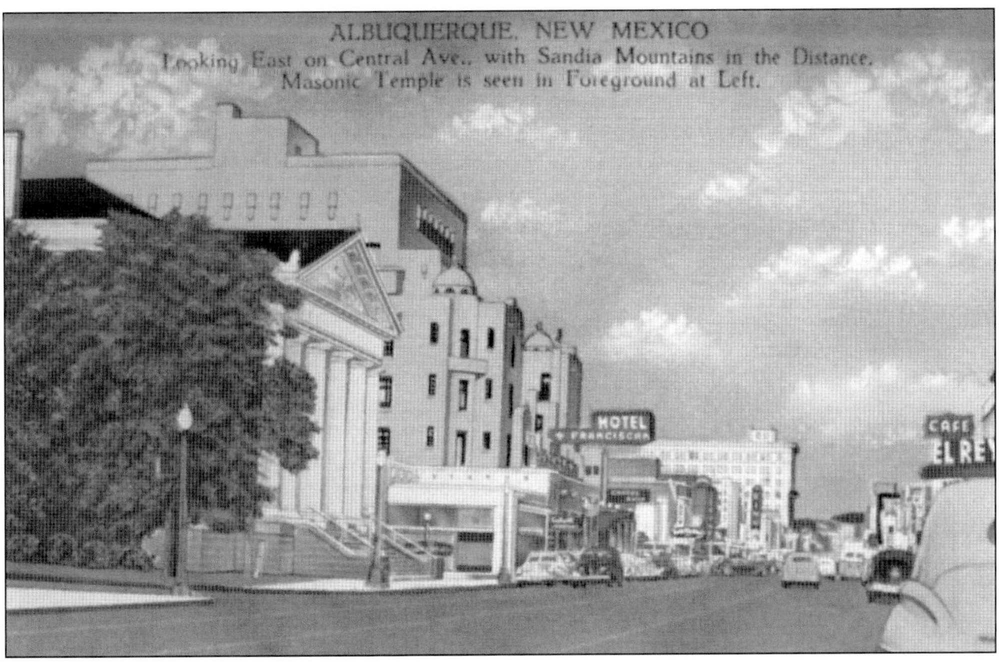

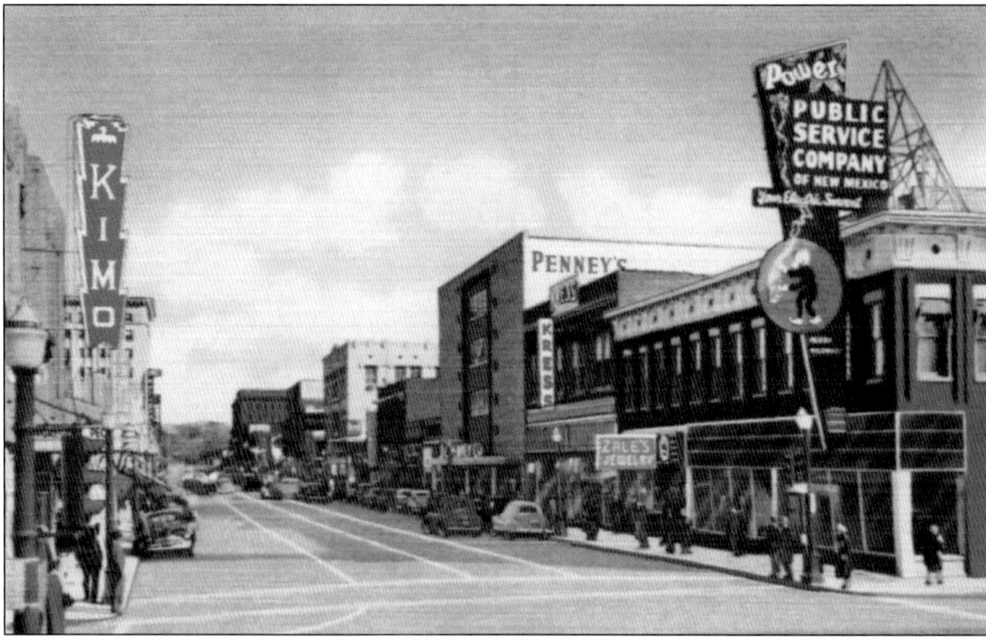

These images show the corner of Central Avenue and Fifth Street. While the dominant buildings at the last corner are gone, this corner is quite recognizable today. The Kimo Theater sign has been recently restored, and the J.C. Penney's building and Public Services building are both still in existence. (Both, courtesy of Nancy Tucker.)

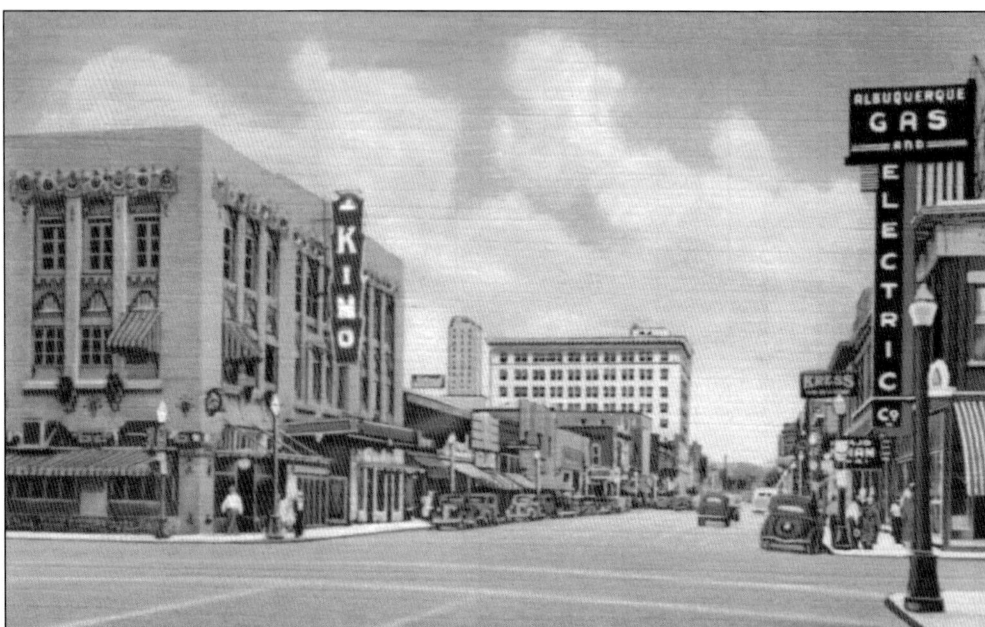

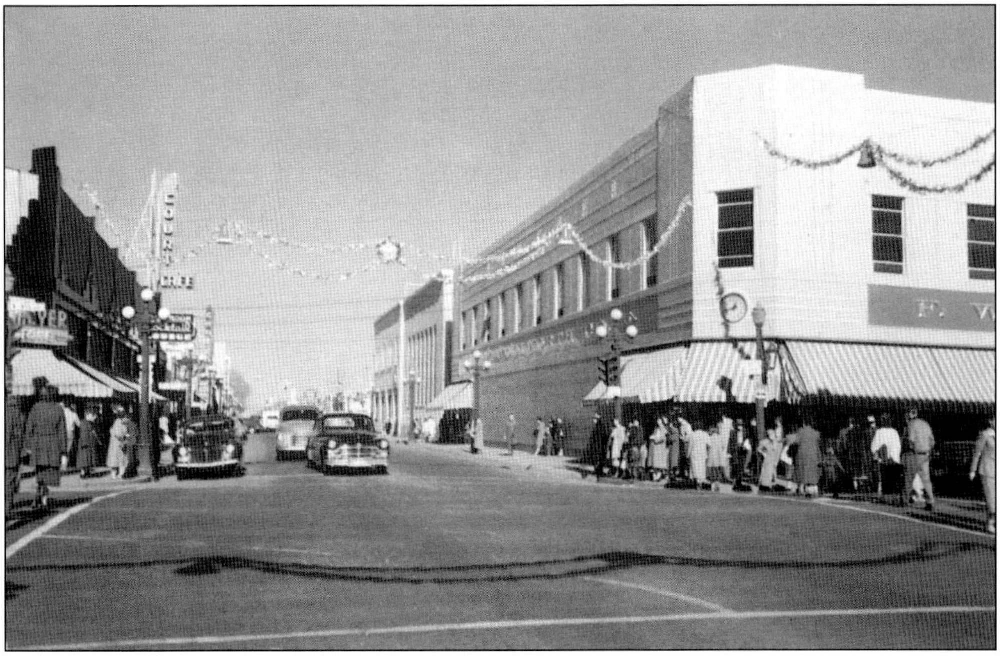

These last two scenes show the corner of Central Avenue and Fourth Street. The above view is looking north up Fourth Street, and the scene below is looking south down the road. Fourth Street is north of Central Avenue and is now a pedestrian street, with the Woolworth building still on the corner. The Court Café only wore its lovely Art Deco facade during the 1930s. (Both, courtesy of Nancy Tucker.)

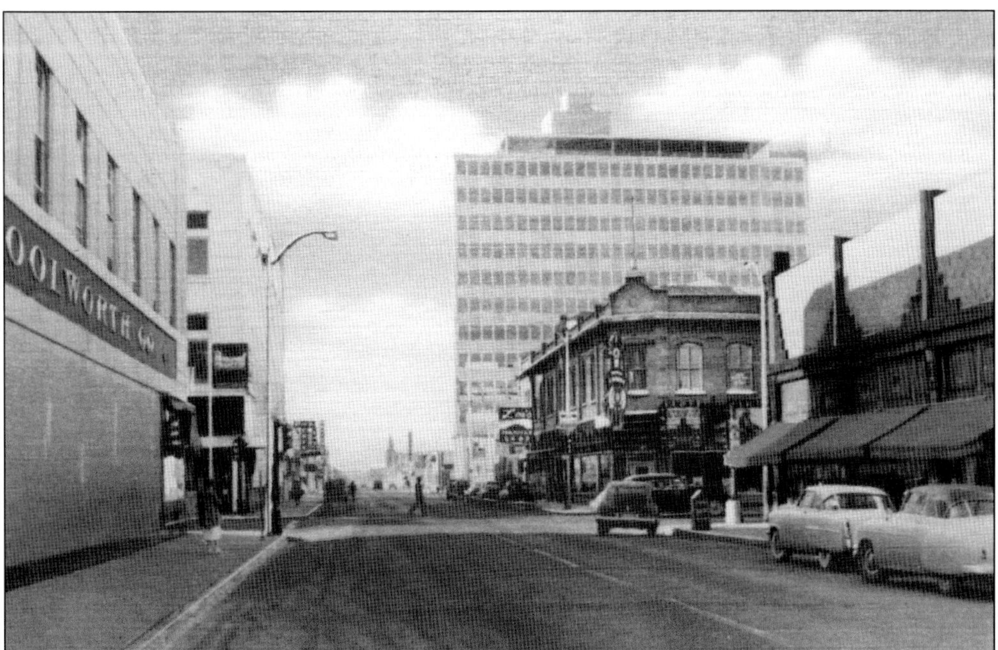

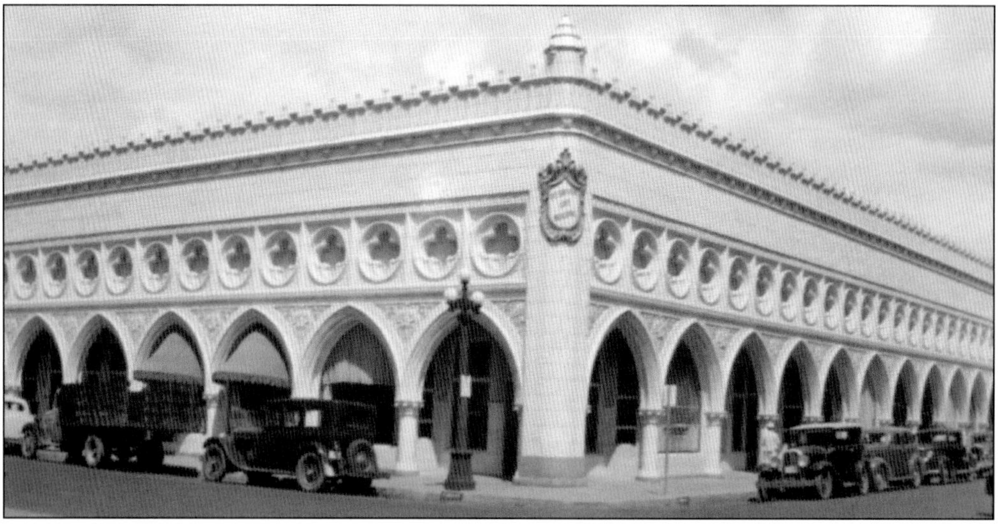

In 1917, the Occidental Insurance Company decided to erect a Doges Place at the northeast corner of Third Street and Gold Avenue. English critic John Ruskin was a favorite author of architect Henry Trost and a great fan of Venice; perhaps Ruskin was the inspiration for this building. Trost had worked in Louis Sullivan's office in Chicago, and a look at the leaves between the arches shows Sullivan's influence. Here is a little taste of Venice by way of Chicago in Albuquerque. (Courtesy of Nancy Tucker.)

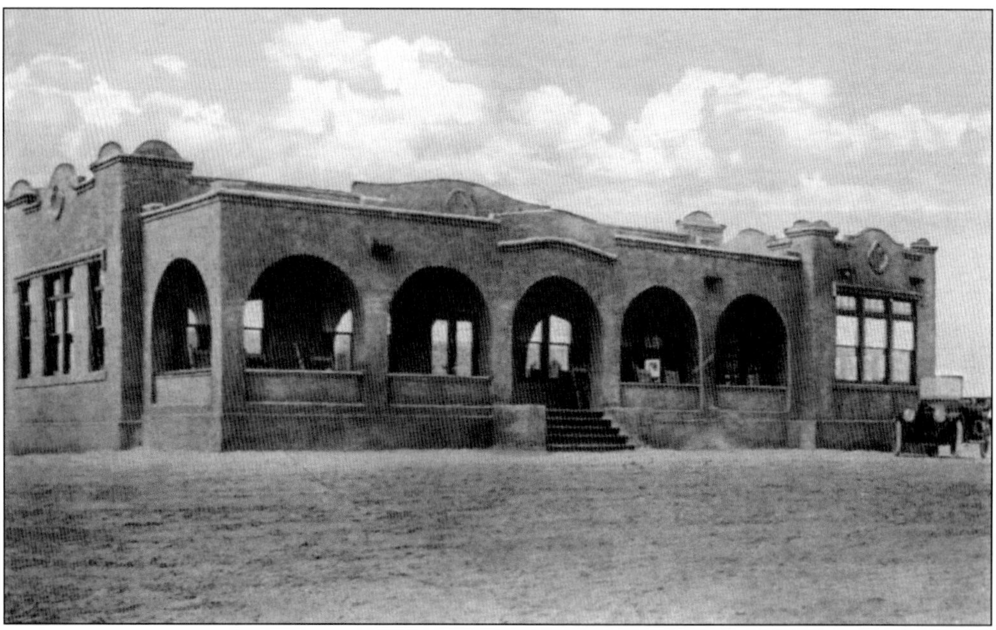

Contrast the arches of Doge with the Mission arches of the Albuquerque County Club. This is likely the first clubhouse built in 1914 in the Mission Revival style. Information about the designer was not found; however, it is typical of a number of buildings of the period. (Courtesy of Nancy Tucker.)

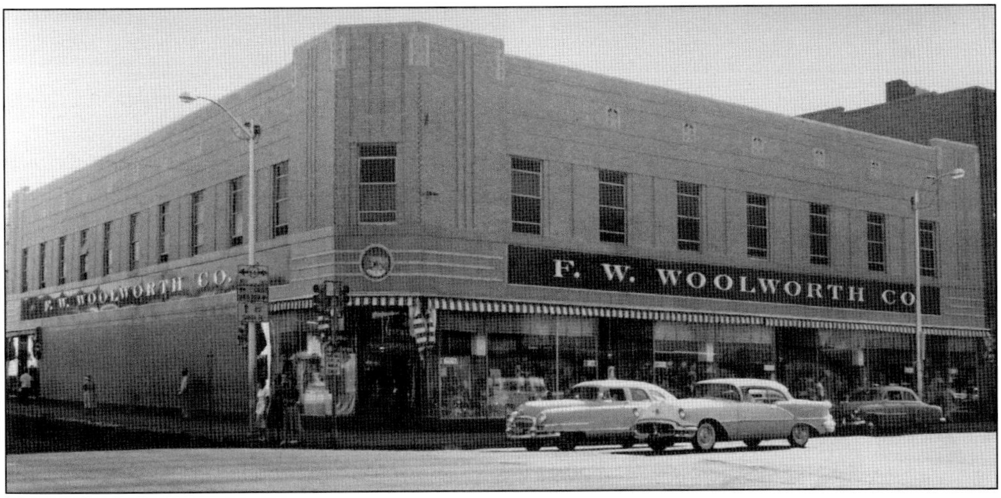

Albuquerque's F.W. Woolworth store was at the northeast corner of Fourth Street and Central Avenue and designed in the early 1940s by Joseph B. Burwinkle, a local architect. However, it is a variation of a standard company design in yellow brick. Its design is rather severe, except for the floral Deco terra-cotta panels near the top. Many similar buildings, some with more terra-cotta trim, are found throughout the United States and Canada. The streetscape postcard of this intersection also shows the Court Café at the lower left, and farther down the street some of the Hilton Hotel and First National Bank are visible. (Both, courtesy of Nancy Tucker.)

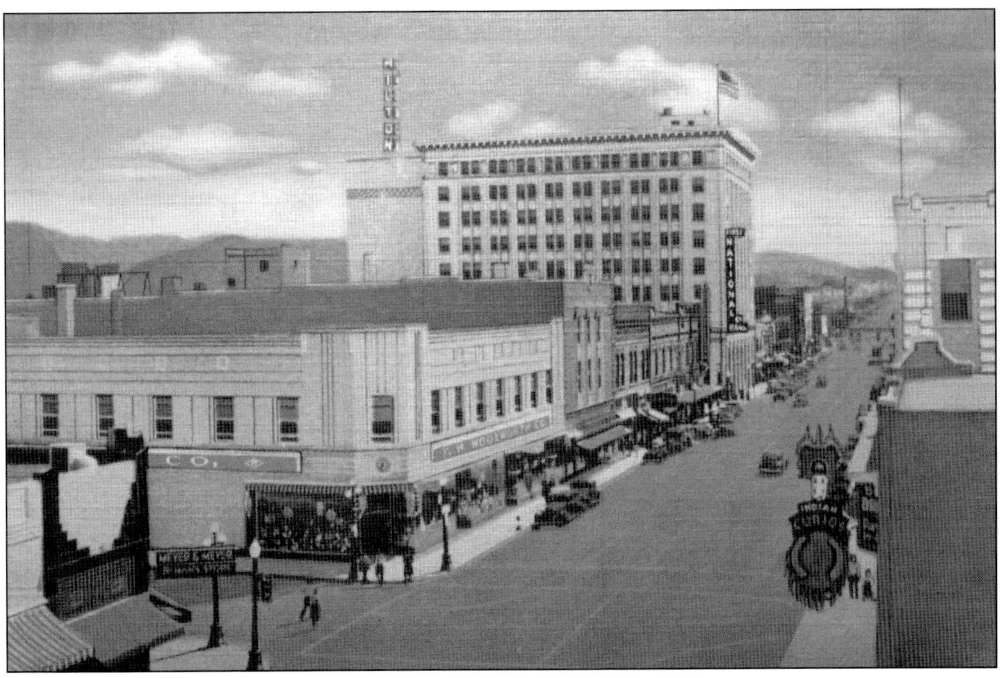

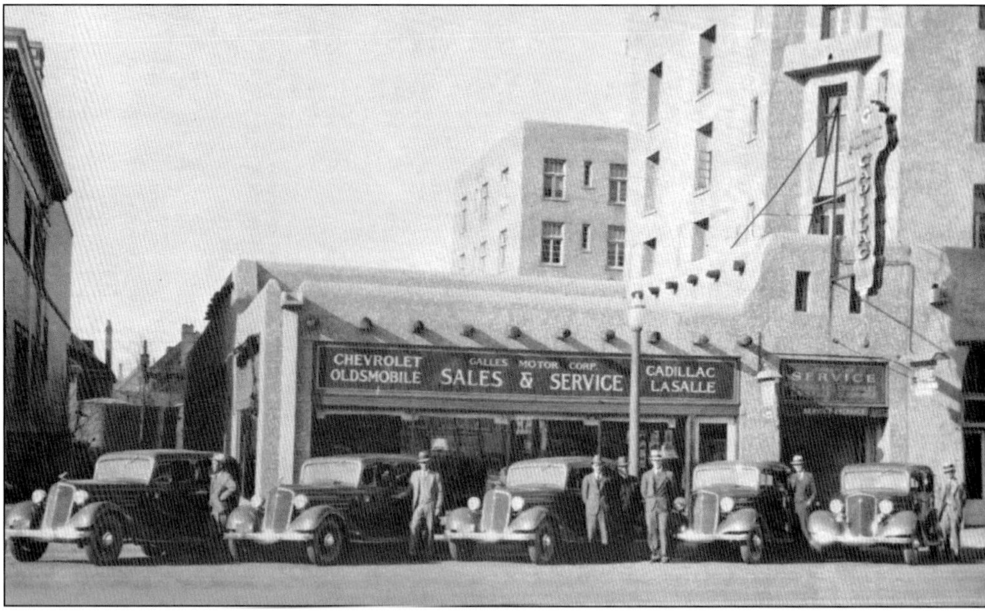

While Art Deco Streamline themes tend to dominate many automobile-related buildings of the 1920s and 1930s, there were some exceptions. This Pueblo Revival building was probably constructed sometime in the 1920s, adjacent to the west side of the Franciscan Hotel. An automobile dealership early on, it later went through a number of retail uses. The heavy beams, *vigas*, and rustic parapet are key characteristics of the style. (Courtesy of Nancy Tucker.)

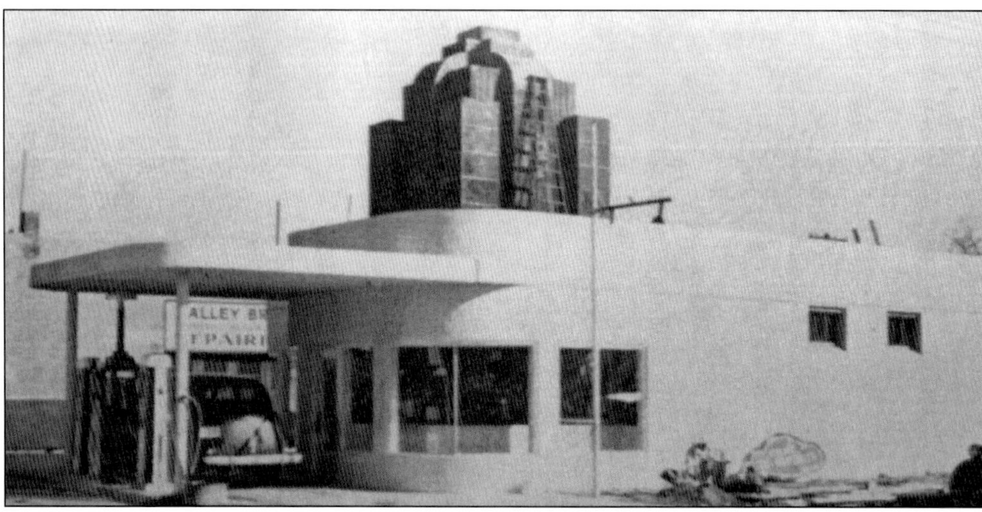

This roof lantern is an Art Deco accoutrement serving no purpose other than identification. There is evidence that the same lantern shape was once on three contemporary Albuquerque service stations. The example here, dated 1939, is on Talley Brother's Standard service station at the corner of North Fourth Street and New York Avenue (a now nonexistent address). A second example was at 1717–1729 Central Avenue, and a third lives on at the northwest corner of Carlisle Boulevard and Central Avenue. (Courtesy of Nancy Tucker.)

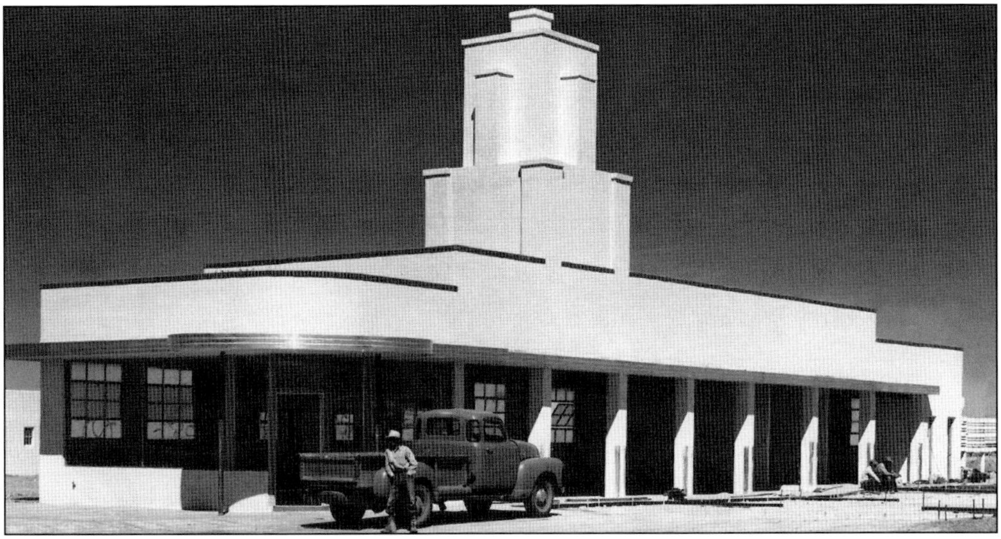

Here are two examples of Streamline Moderne forms. The above photograph is the "new" Jones Ford Motor Company branch dealership on Lomas Boulevard. This picture dates from 1951, although the building's design is clearly a throwback to the original 1939 Jones Dealership on Central Avenue. The Carothers and Fuller service station was at 320 East Central Avenue and dates from the late 1930s. It is now the period-themed Standard Diner. (Above, courtesy of the Museum of Albuquerque; below, courtesy of Nancy Tucker.)

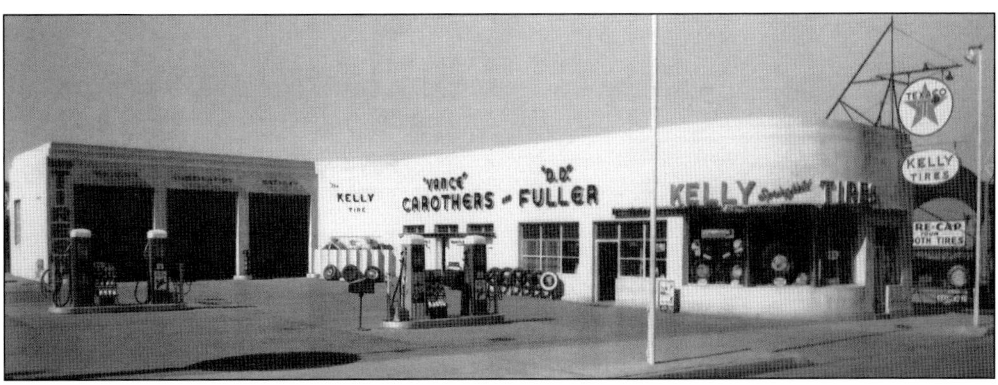

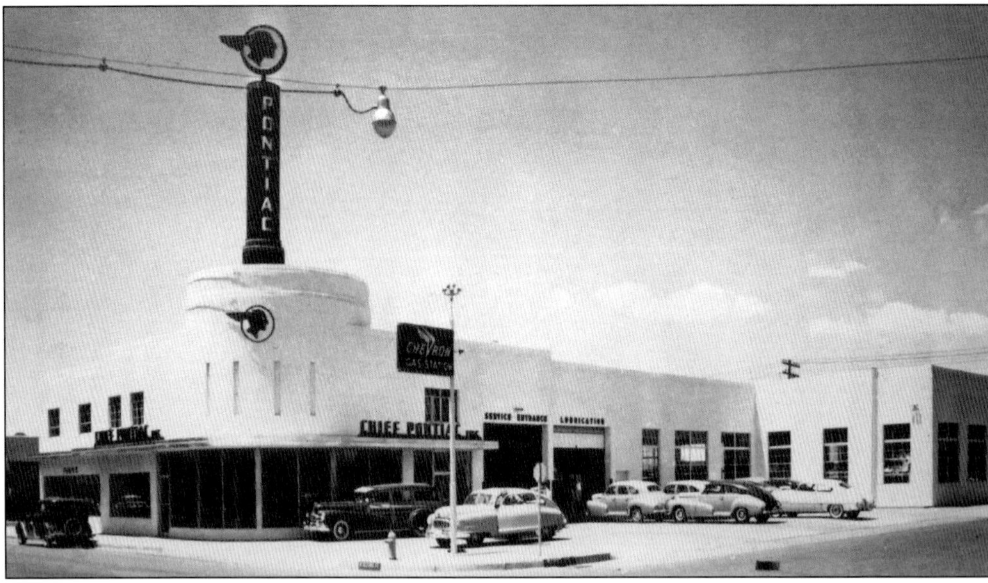

Streamline Moderne could also take on decidedly vertical components. Chief Pontiac, Inc., was located at 625 North Second Street. Its corner tower sports a column topped by the iconic Pontiac emblem. The building appears to date from the mid- to late 1930s and no longer exists. Fortunately, the Excelsior Laundry at the southeast corner of Second and Roma Streets still exists. It has a Moderne tower sign flanked by glass bricks integral to the building's front facade. (Both, courtesy of Nancy Tucker.)

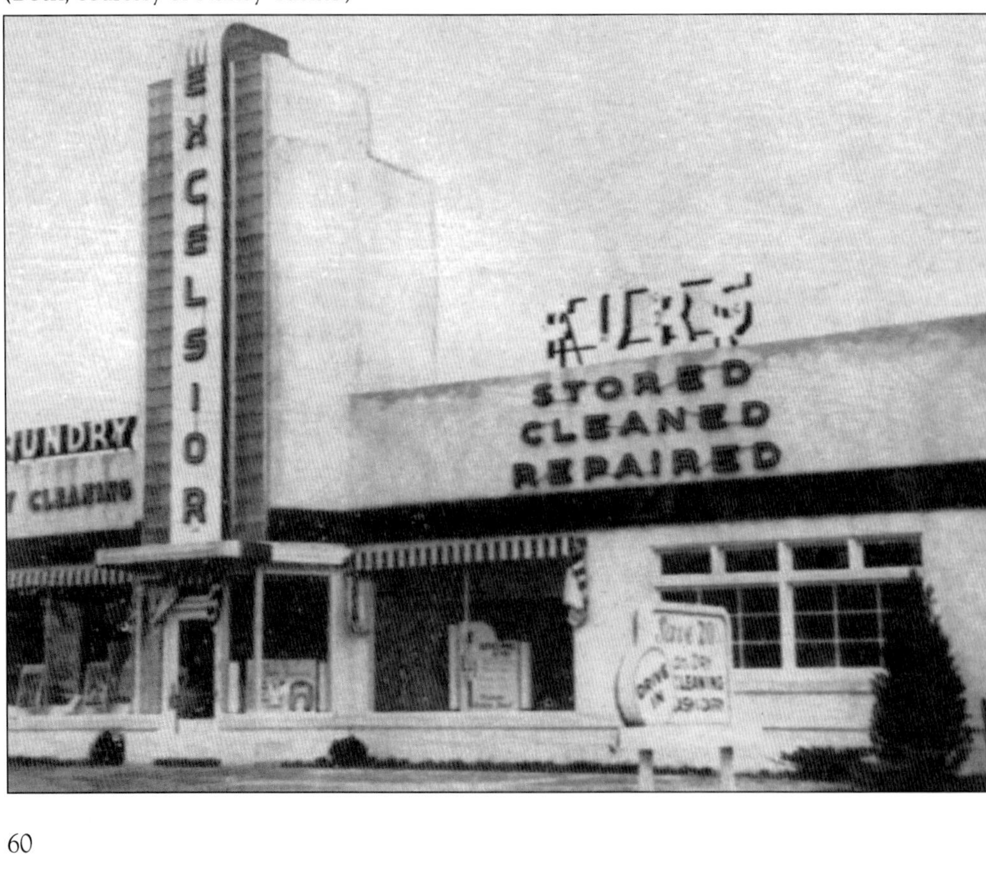

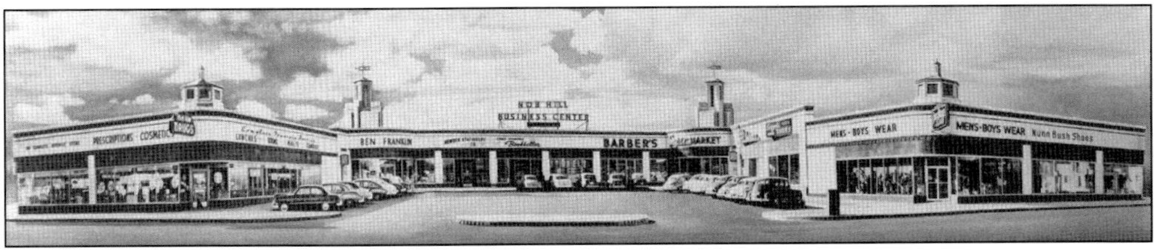

The Nob Hill Shopping Center, located at the Southwest corner of Central Avenue and Carlisle Boulevard, is a tribute to the automobile and is recognized as one of the best remaining examples of a 1940s-era, automobile-oriented shopping center in America. It was developed by Robert B. Waggoman in 1947 and designed by local architect Louis Hesselden, who also designed several 1930s and 1940s additions to the old Albuquerque High School. The Nob Hill Shopping Center's Moderne design elements incorporate a brick coping reminiscent of Territorial styling, described for the Hilton Hotel on page 102. (Both, courtesy of Nancy Tucker.)

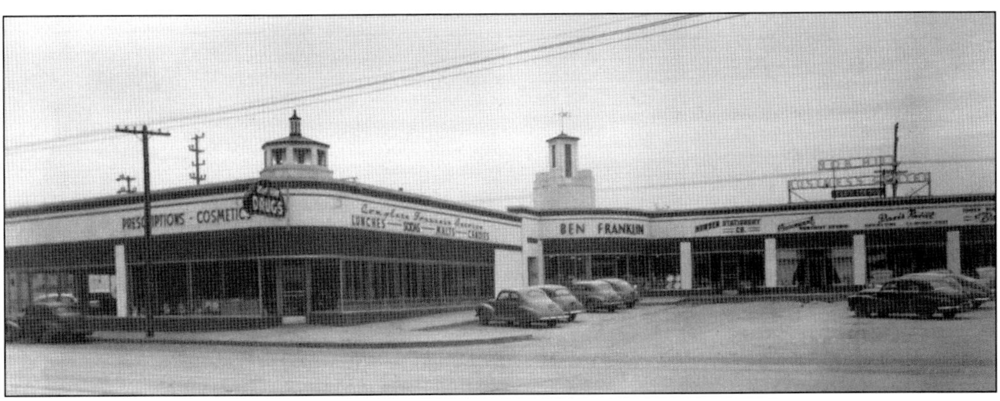

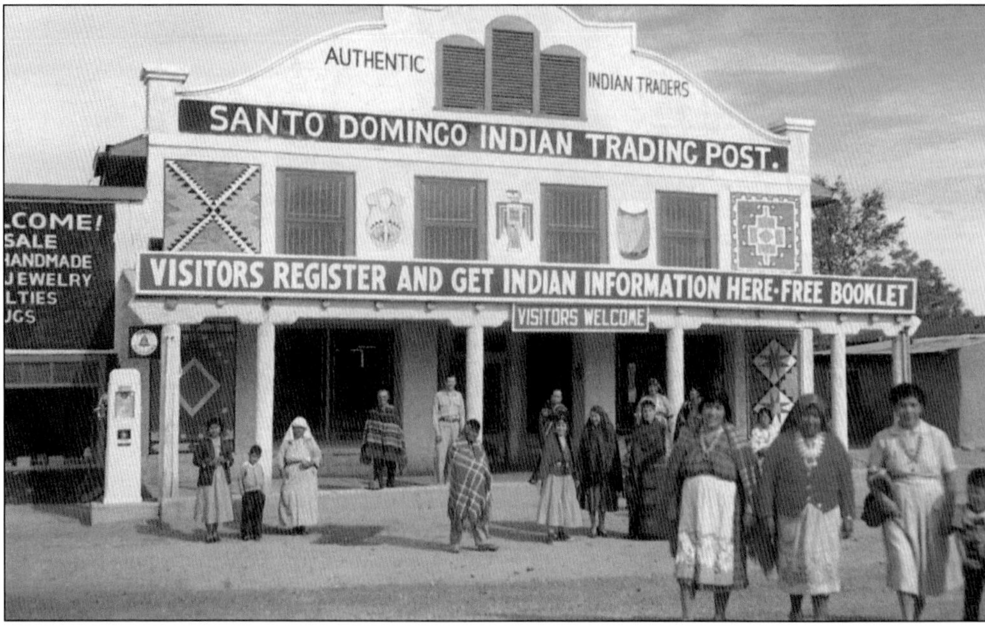
AUTHENTIC
INDIAN TRADERS
SANTO DOMINGO INDIAN TRADING POST.
VISITORS REGISTER AND GET INDIAN INFORMATION HERE·FREE BOOKLET
VISITORS WELCOME

The Seligman family founded the Santo Domingo Trading Post, at Santo Domingo, now Kewa Pueblo, in 1880. The addition shown here was built in 1922. Located adjacent to a rail stop and Route 66 (until the highway was realigned in 1937), the building's Mission Revival architecture is similar to that of other Atchison, Topeka & Santa Fe structures. In 2001, the structure burned; however, there are plans for it to be rebuilt. (Courtesy of Dr. Ted Jojola.)

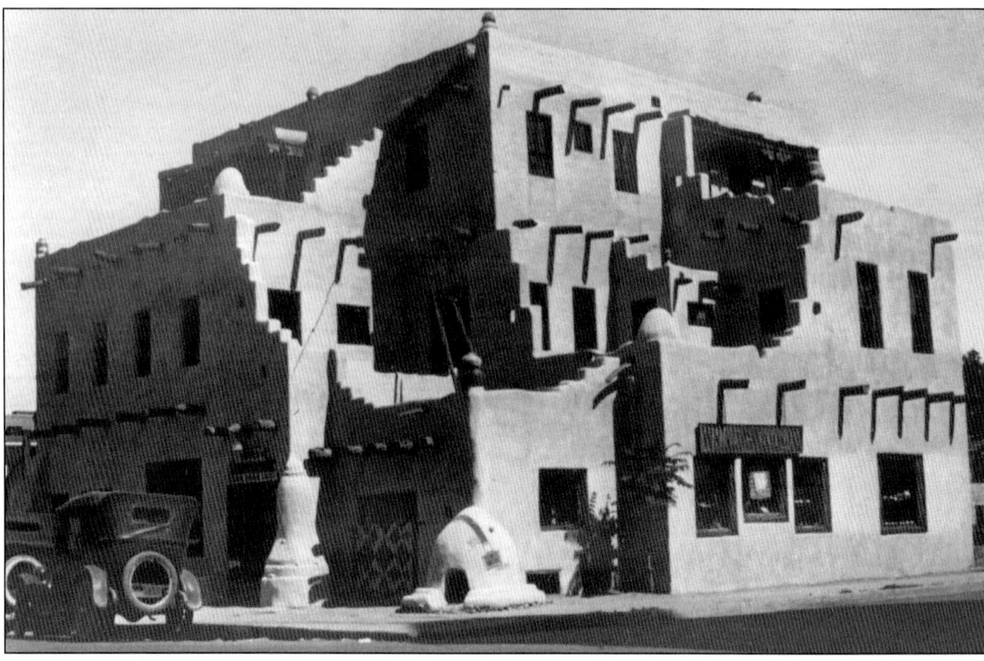

Wright's Trading Post was located in this pseudo pueblo, which was built in 1920, at the corner of Third Street and Gold Avenue until the structure was demolished in 1958. The interior is said to have been especially impressive with huge pine beams, a 10-foot-high adobe fireplace, and a reconstruction of a Navajo sweathouse. (Courtesy of Nancy Tucker.)

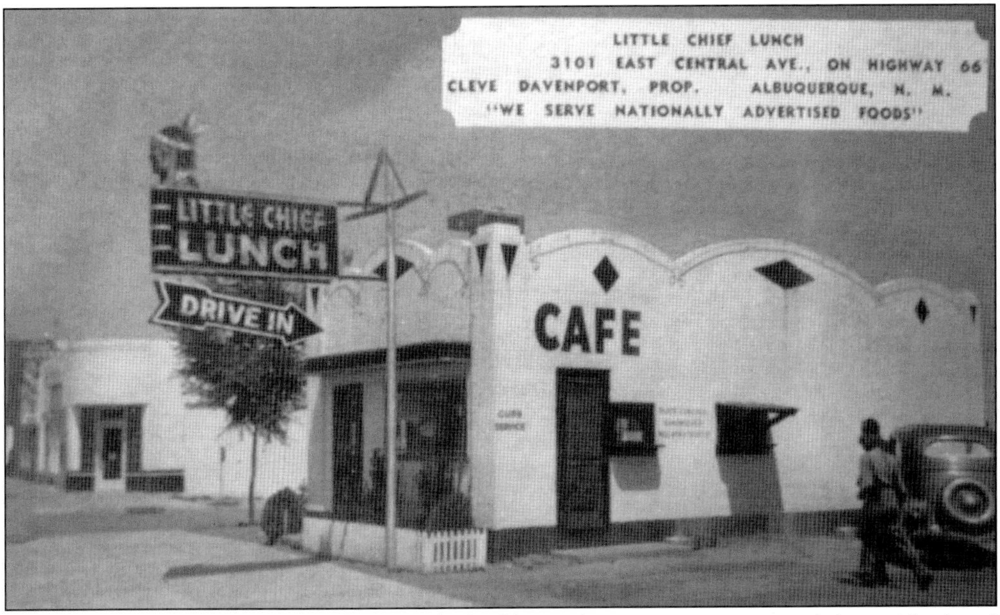
LITTLE CHIEF LUNCH
3101 EAST CENTRAL AVE., ON HIGHWAY 66
CLEVE DAVENPORT, PROP. ALBUQUERQUE, N. M.
"WE SERVE NATIONALLY ADVERTISED FOODS"
LITTLE CHIEF
LUNCH
DRIVE IN
CAFE

While this book has concentrated on grander buildings, there were numerous stylish neighborhood cafés and small businesses. Some of these exhibit a strong regional character, while others aspire to be thoroughly modern. Here are two examples: both have Deco signs typical of the 1930s. The Little Chief has a Mission Revival feel with its arched parapet, painted diamonds, and triangles. The National Bakery and Cafeteria is up-to-date with no regional influence; note the zigzag facade to the right. (Above, courtesy of Nancy Tucker; below, courtesy of the Museum of Albuquerque.)

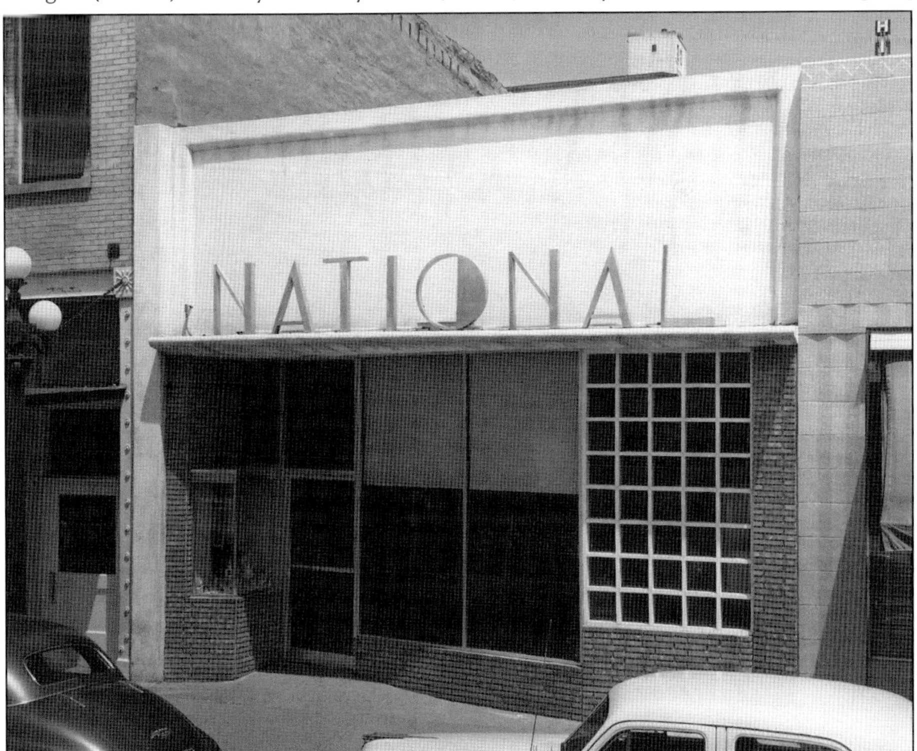

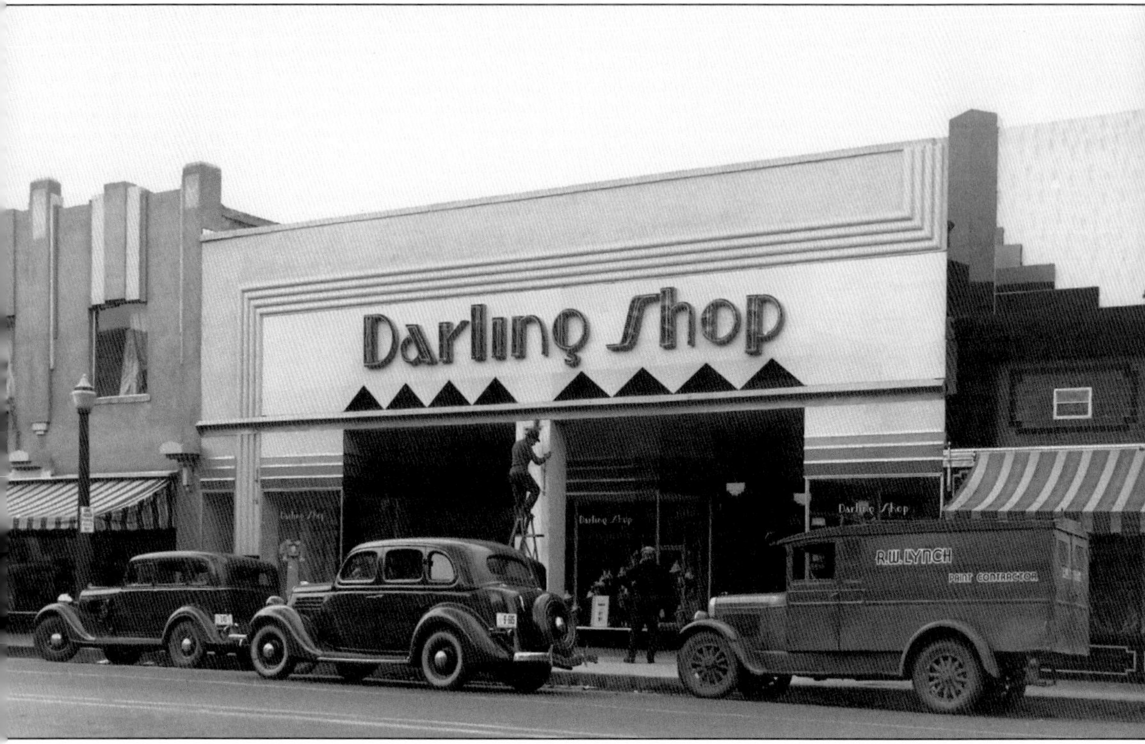

What a shame it is that this 1933 streetscape, located at the north side of Central Avenue and west of Fourth Street, no longer exists. The western end of the Court Café building, see opposite image, is visible on the right. The Darling Shop was a woman's clothing store. Does this picture show the final stages of a new facade? Are the black glass triangles a nod to regional influences? The 1920s vertical facade to the left belongs to a unidentified retail store. The automobiles appear to be Chrysler products, and the truck is a Mack. (Courtesy of the Museum of Albuquerque.)

Here is the Court Café in its fully Art Deco splendor, a look the building apparently only had during the 1930s. Angular towers at the corner and along the tiled parapet are clad in black Carrara glass panels, providing vertical accents to the facade. The spaces between look to be tile. Colored glass fills in the transoms with black tile below. (Courtesy of Nancy Tucker.)

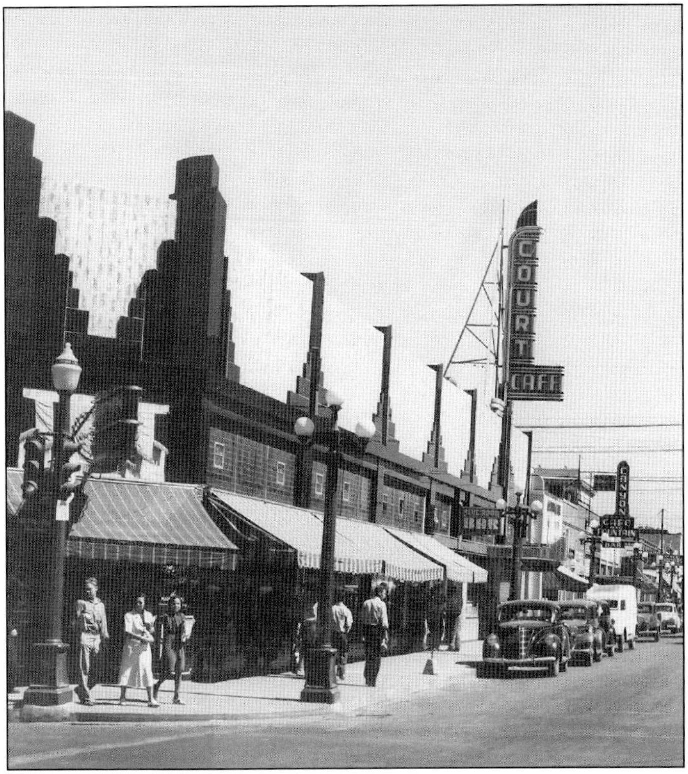

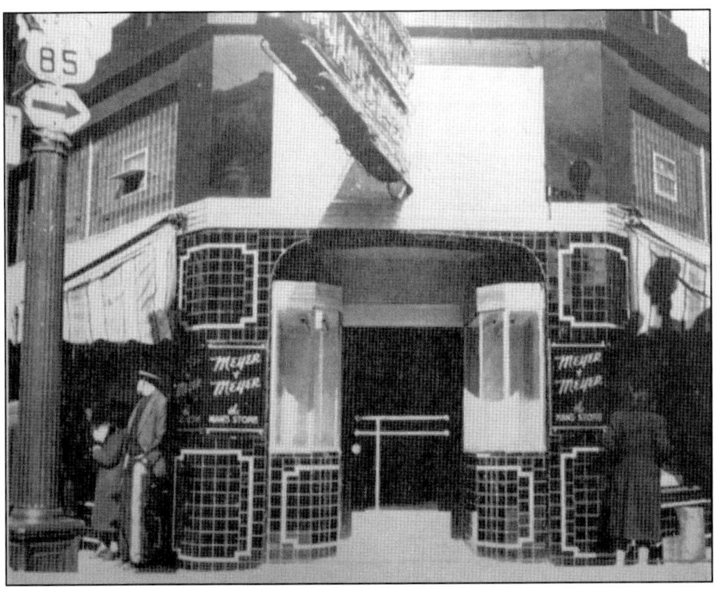

The Court Café building was at the northeast corner of Central Avenue and Fourth Street. Meyer & Meyer men's store occupied the corner with the café and bar entrance off Fourth Street. The building has been remodeled a number of times. Unfortunately, nothing remains of its 1930s Deco facade. (Courtesy of Nancy Tucker.)

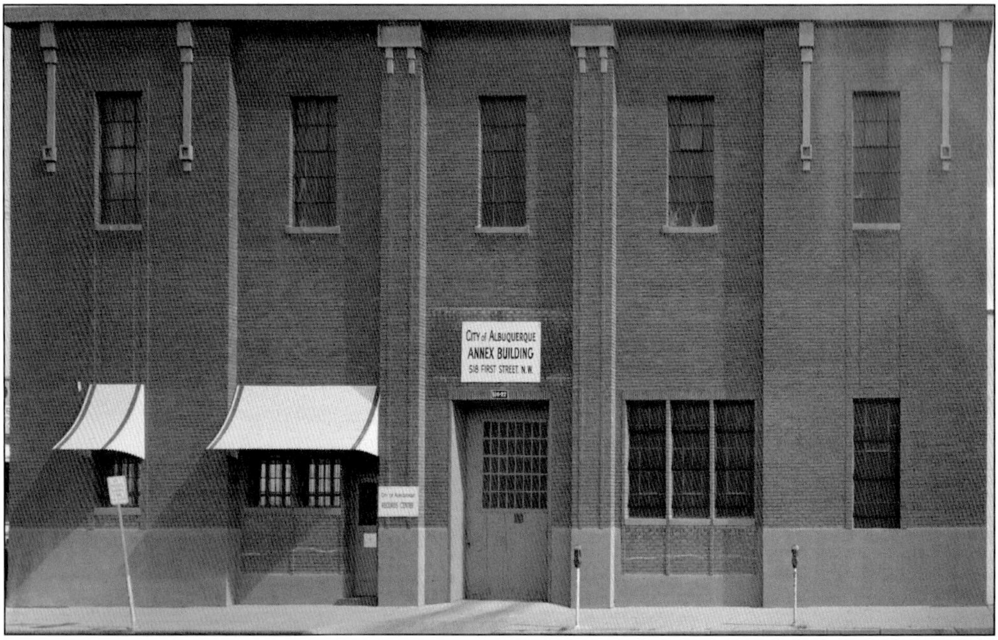

The Wool Warehouse at 516–522 First Street is a simple brick box with some interesting Egyptian Revival detailing. Inside, 36 massive lotus blossom capital columns support the roof. The structure was built in 1928 and was designed by Tjalke Charles Gaastra (1879–1937), a Dutch architect who moved to New Mexico in 1918 and is known principally for his Spanish-Pueblo Revival buildings in Santa Fe. (Courtesy of Nancy Tucker.)

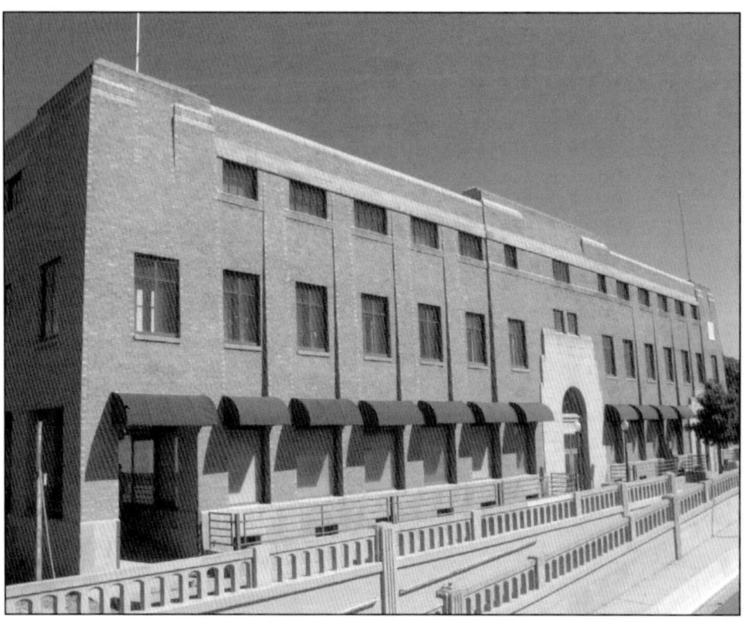

The Springer Transfer Company office and warehouse, located at 121 Tijeras, was designed in 1930 by local architect George Williamson. It is an example of Meso-American massing translated into a modern composition. The entrances, with their stepped corbels, are distinctly Mayan, as are the Greek key designs. (Author's collection.)

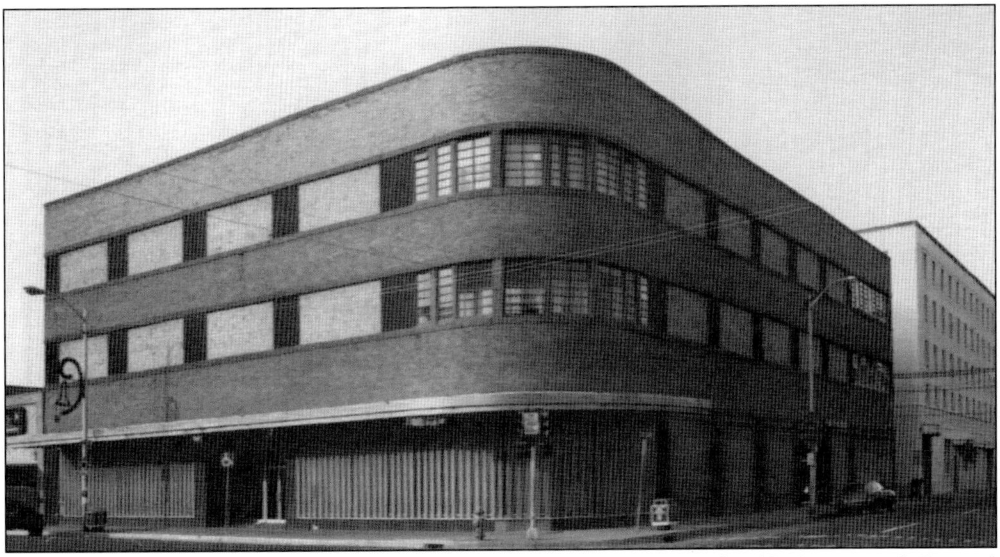

The 1937 Streamline Moderne Lovelace building at the corner of Fifth Street and Central Avenue is the first of three modernist buildings by John Gaw Meem included in this book. The buff-colored brick building was constructed in three installments for Dr. William R. Lovelace, a prominent Albuquerque physician. In 1953, the building was leased to Sears. (Courtesy of the UNM CSWR John Gaw Meem Collection.)

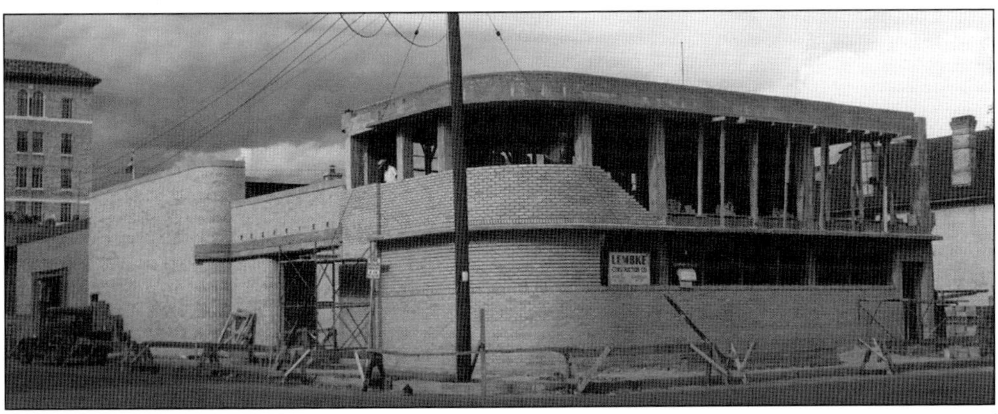

KOB radio station built new Streamline Moderne studios in 1937 at the northeast corner of Fifth Street and Gold Avenue in the same year as the Lembke house (see pages 16 and 114). The architect is not known, but a Lembke Construction Co. sign is clearly visible. While this building no longer survives, there is a similar tan brick Streamline structure on Gold Avenue, a block to the west. (Courtesy of the Albuquerque City Planning Department.)

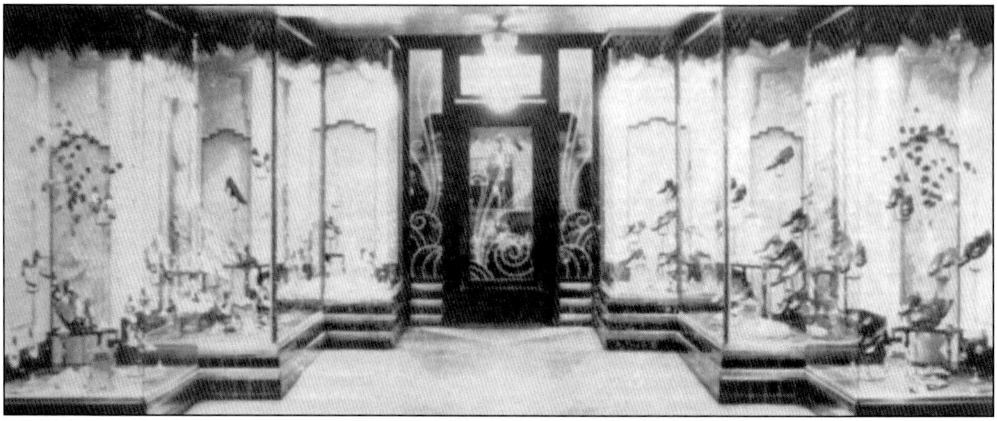

The Paris Shoe Store was located at 307 West Central Avenue. This advertising photograph from 1937 is illustrative of a thoroughly modern retail storefront, with black tile and curvilinear metal-door grating. This makes an interesting contrast with Maisel's storefront (see page 77) from two years later. (Courtesy of the Albuquerque City Planning Department.)

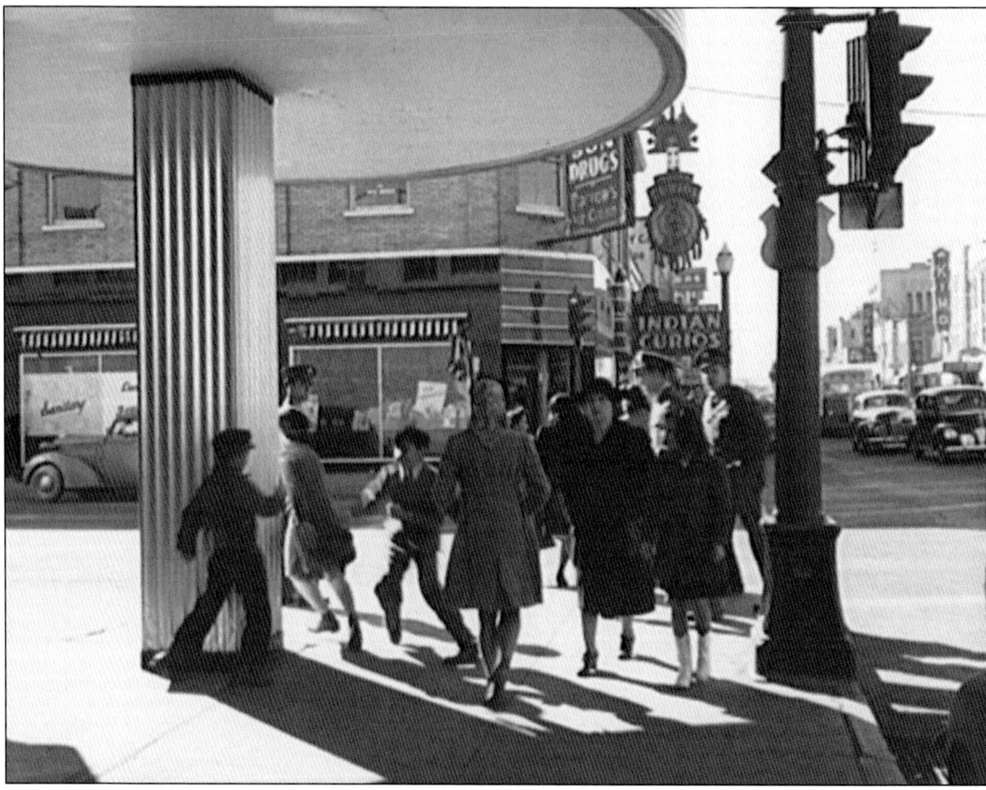

The Rosenwald Building at the southeast corner of Fourth Street and Central Avenue was designed by Trost &Trost and built in 1910. Sometime in the 1930s, McLellan's Department store added a rather incongruous freestanding Deco cover over its corner street entry. This photograph is from the early 1940s. Note the second Maisel's location, at this time still an Indian store, across the street. (See pages 72 and 73.) (Courtesy of the Albuquerque City Planning Department.)

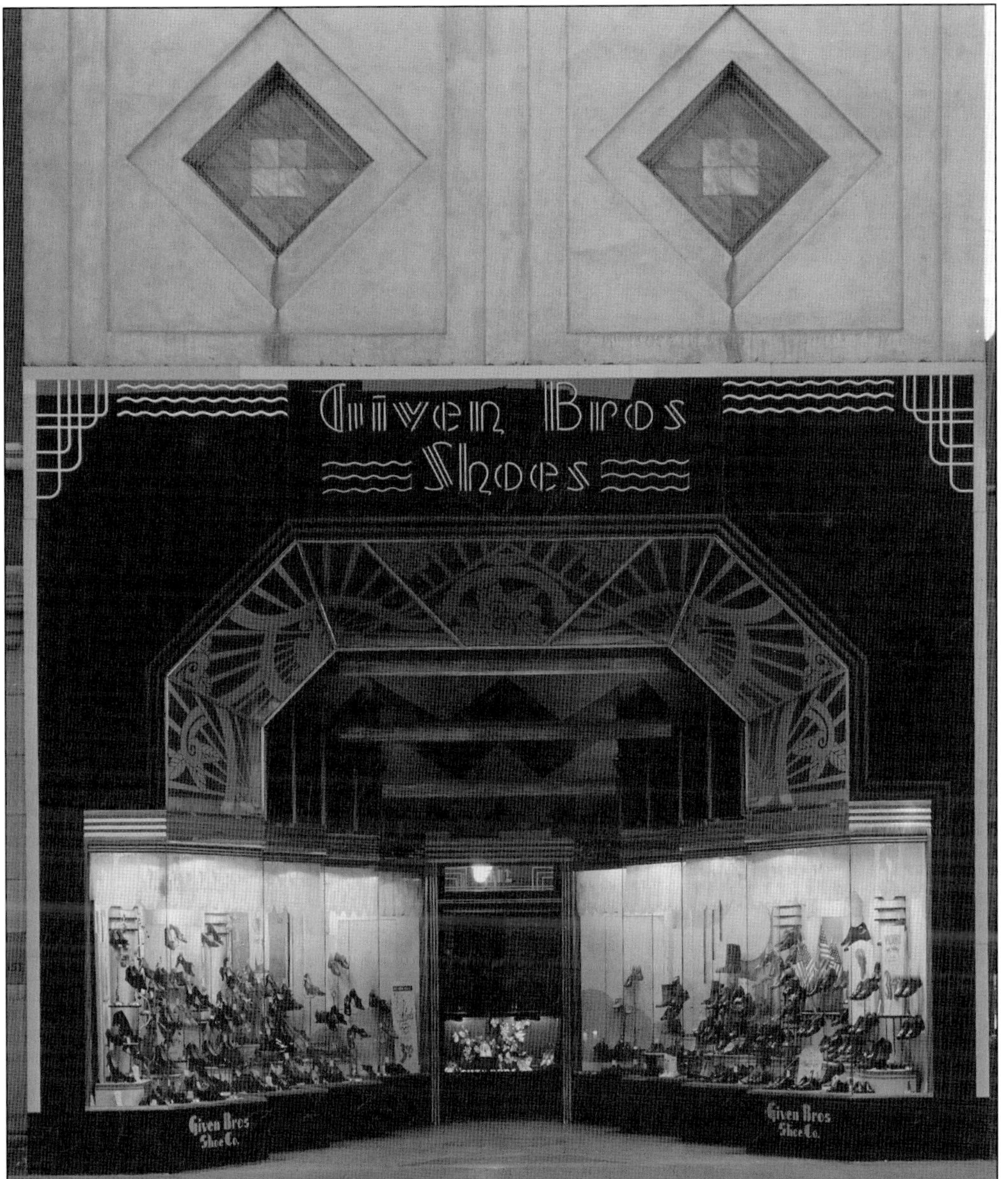

Across the street from the Paris Shoe Store was Given Bros. Shoes. This store was a fixture in downtown Albuquerque for many years and, keeping up with the time, modernized its storefront several times. Here is the store as it appeared in the later 1930s and 1940s with striking Deco-etched black Carrara glass panels and diamond-shaped, stained-glass windows on the second level. The building now houses the Library Bar and Grill, but the beautiful Given storefront is long gone. (Courtesy of the Albuquerque City Planning Department.)

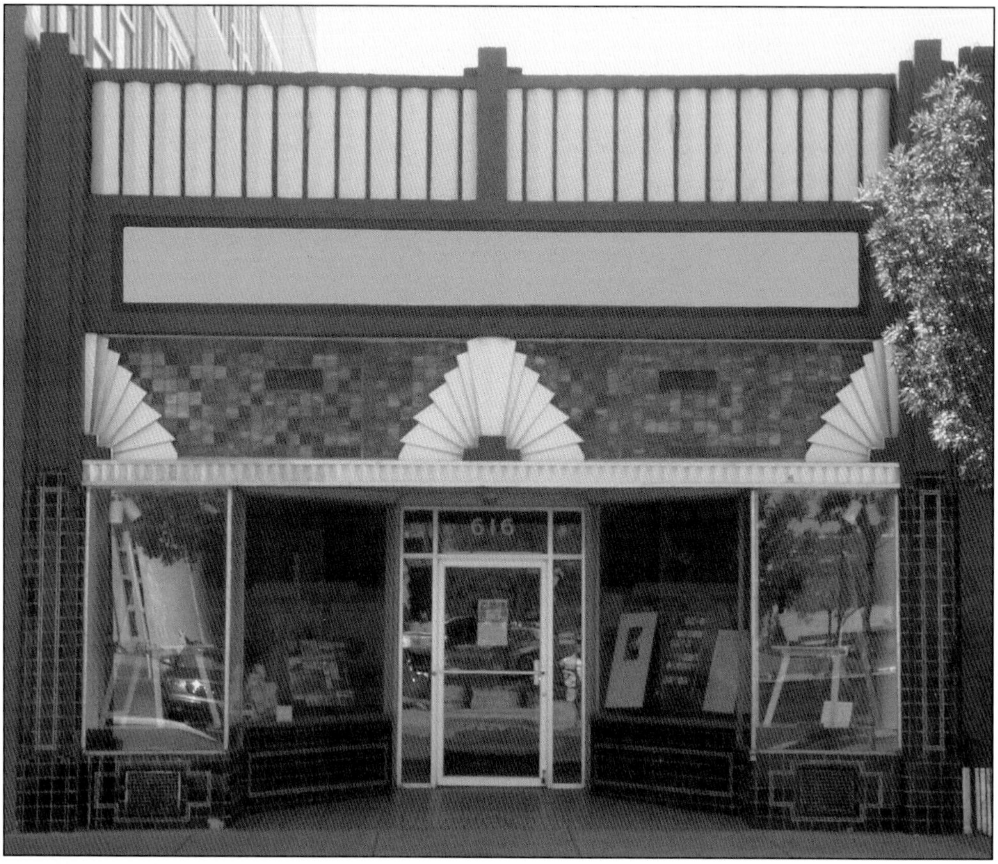

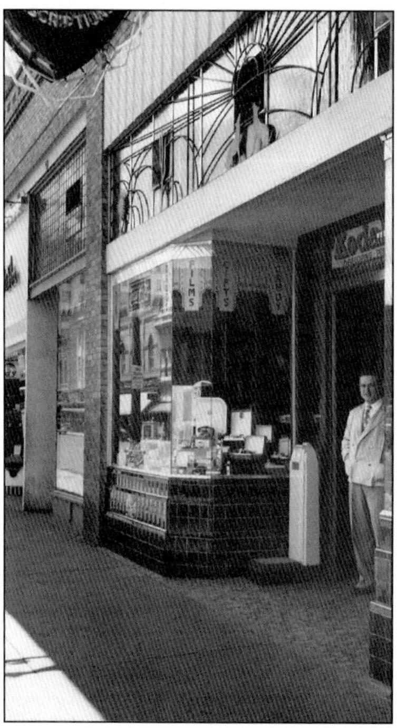

At 616 Central Avenue is this Deco "sunburst." Green and brown opalescent glass set off the metal sunburst and side fans. Black and green glazed tile flank the entry. From 1933 until 1965, this was the location of Fremont's Fine Food, founded by Chinese emigrant Edward Gaw Tang, who came to Albuquerque in 1918 to start a new life. Fremont's was the premier speciality food store in town for many years and continues to this day under fourth-generation ownership as a catering business. The building dates from the early 20th century, while this front is early 1930s. In the early 1970s, the building was occupied by Wright's Trading Post, and it is now a Holocaust Museum. To the left is Arrow Drugs on Central Avenue in 1938, with a similar facade to that of 616 Central Avenue. The metal open-work above the entrance is true Coyote Deco! (Above, author's collection; left, courtesy of the Museum of Albuquerque.)

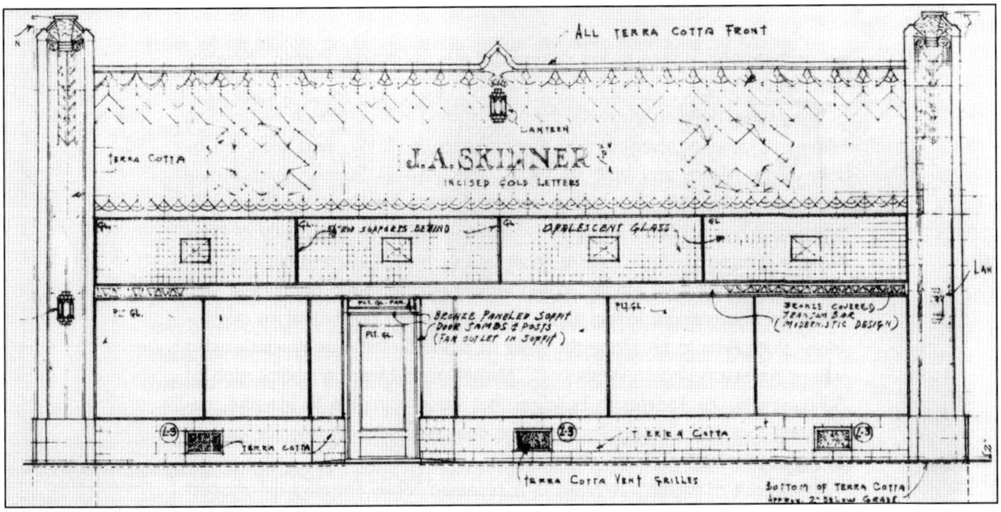

Skinner Grocery is at the southwest corner of Eighth Street and Central Avenue; see a photograph of the front of the building on page 15. The design is by architect Albert William Boehning (1891–1962), who began his career as a cabinetmaker, worked for Trost & Trost, and then struck out on his own in 1925. This building was constructed in 1931 and is one of the few he designed in an overtly Art Deco style, as most of his designs are Mission and Spanish Colonial Revival. Decorative glazed terra-cotta tiles with green and white stained-glass windows, coupled with the interplay of vertical and horizontal lines, make this an especially good example of Art Deco. It is interesting to compare with the Fremont Food storefront facade shown opposite. (Above, courtesy of the UNM CSWR; below, courtesy of the Museum of Albuquerque.)

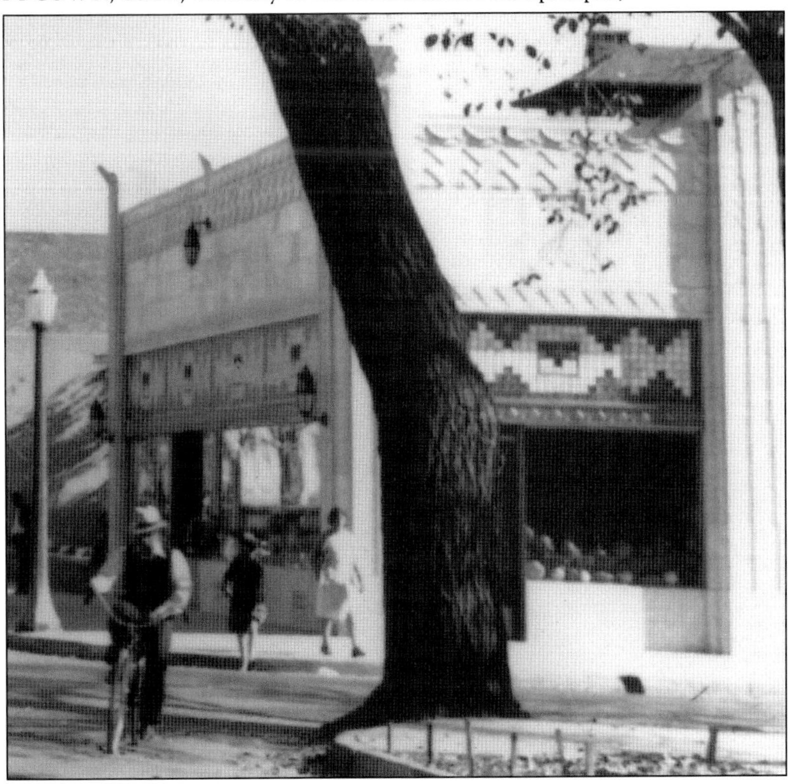

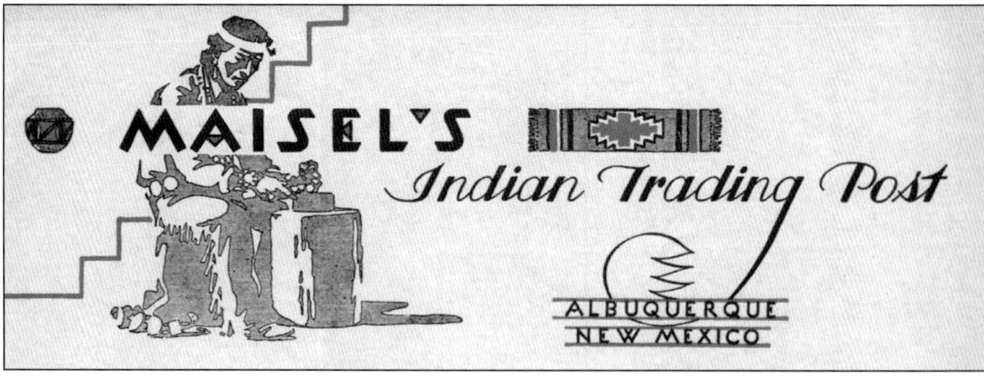

Maurice Maisel first opened his Indian store in 1923 at the southwest corner of Central Avenue and First Street, across from the Alvarado Hotel. Later, the store moved into the Yrisarri Building, which is shown here at 400–408 Central Avenue. The ground floor of this Victorian building has been given a modern 1920s black Carrara glass front. Pueblo and Navajo craftsman worked in the store, as Maurice traveled the Southwest in his Model T. Nelson and Winthrop Rockefeller purchased their wedding bands at Maisel's, and in the 1950s, every Shriner in New Mexico wore a turquoise pin from Maisel's commissioned by Sen. Clinton P. Anderson. Although in a brick 19th-century commercial building, the ground floor street frontage was apparently remodeled by Maisel in the early 1920s and echoes the design aesthetic of the later store at 510 Central Avenue. (Both, courtesy of Skip Maisel.)

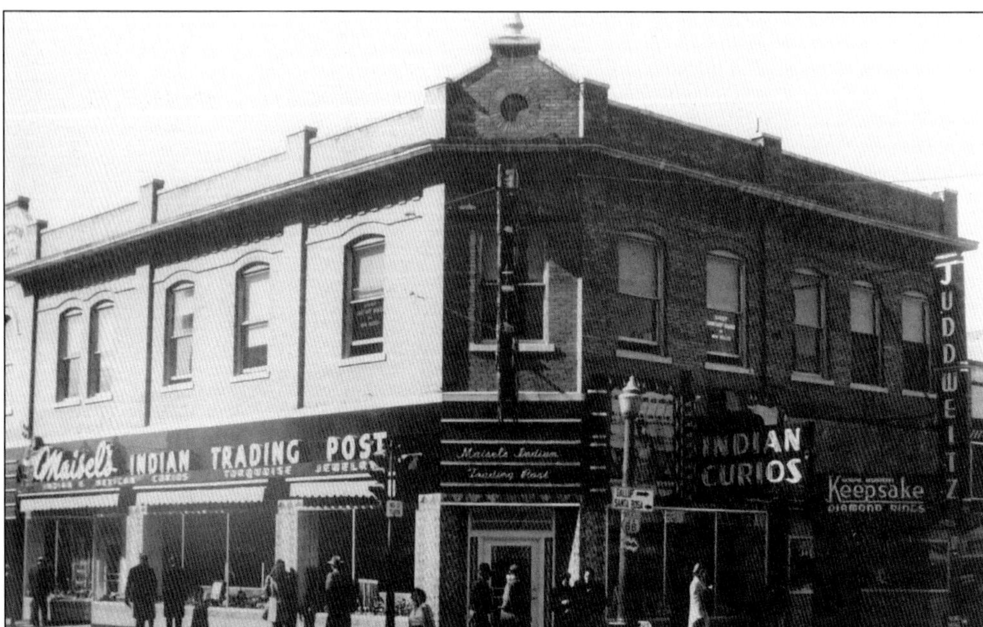

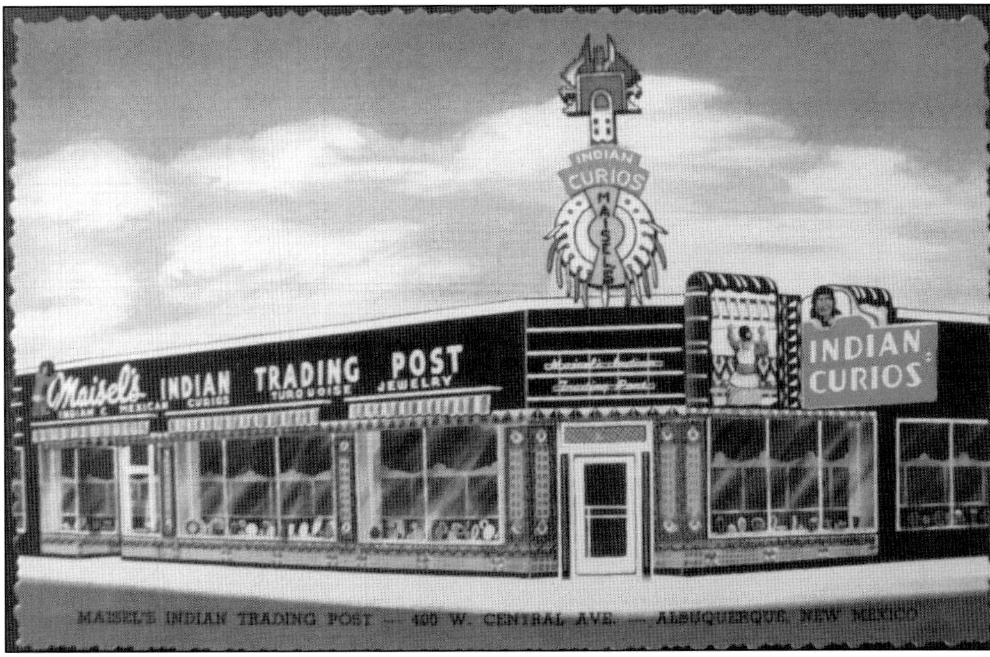

The above postcard is another picture of the original storefront—without the second story! Maisel's employed Native Americans who produced jewelry sold on the premises. There is a large opening in the floor of the store so patrons can view the basement workshop. This photograph shows the cover of one of Maisel's catalogs, probably from the early 1930s, which contains photographs of hundreds of bracelets, earrings, belts, etc., that could be ordered by vendors in bulk. A contract dated 1943 for a jewelry worker states that the pay was 45¢ an hour, standard laborer wage for the time. (Both, courtesy of Skip Maisel.)

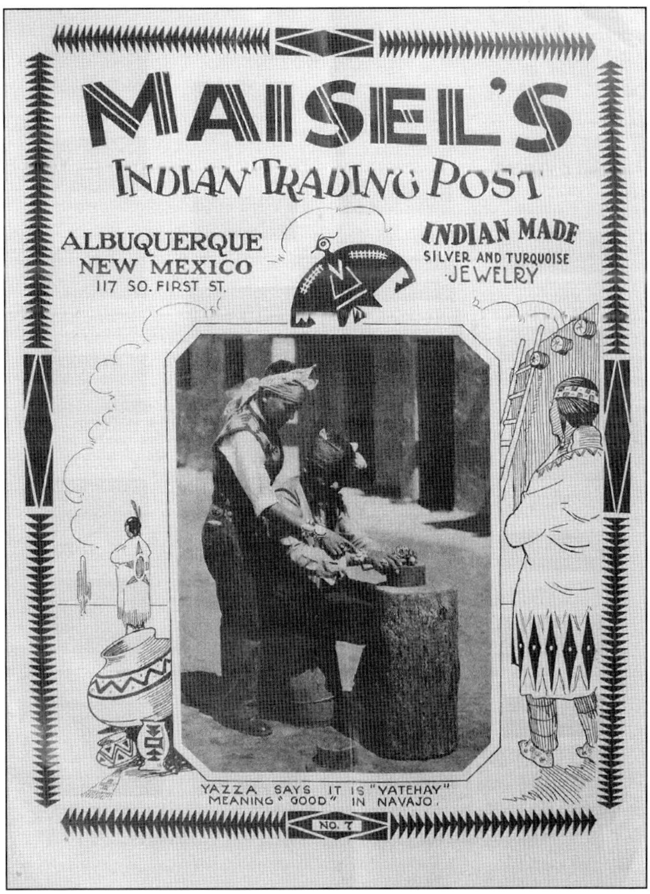

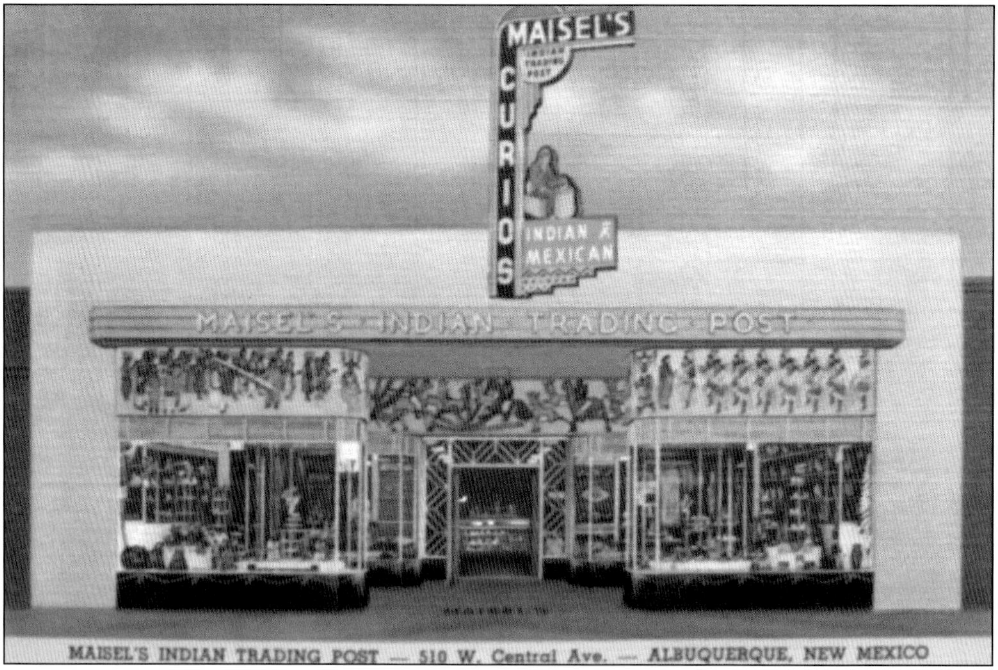

Construction for Maisel's Indian Jewelry and Crafts building at 510 Central Avenue began in 1937, and it opened on June 21, 1939. Architect John Gaw Meem was the principal designer. In this case, however, his client required that the building be "a strictly modern structure using where necessary Indian symbols." A mural created by Pueblo and Navajo artists forms a high band unifying the entry. Cast aluminum molding surrounds the entrance door and evokes Navajo textile designs as well as Pueblo cloud forms often found on pottery. Below, is a concept sketch by Meem that clearly shows the black Carrara glass band with an etched "plumed serpent," called an Awanyu, often found on black Santa Clara and San Ildefonso pottery designs. (Both, courtesy of Skip Maisel.)

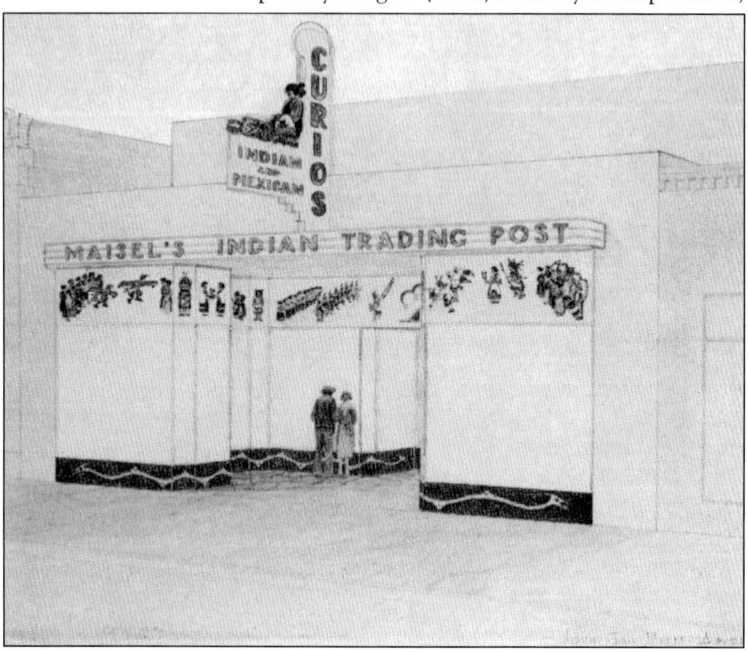

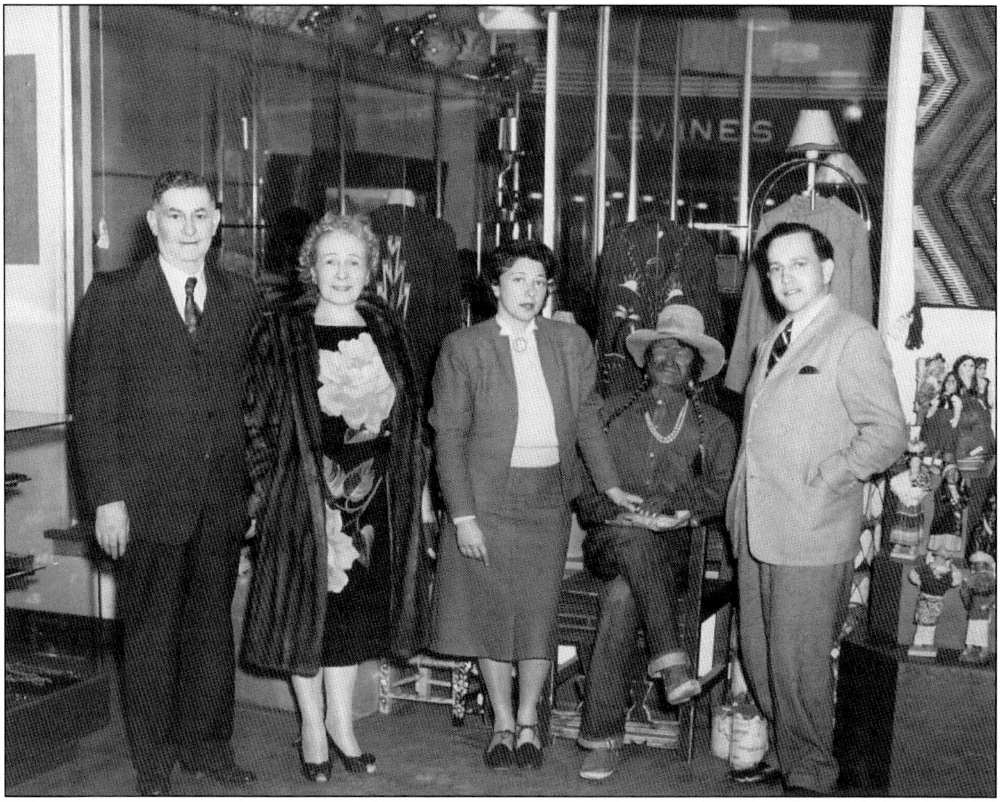

Maurice Maisel, an Austrian immigrant who came to America in 1896 and moved to New Mexico in 1910, began selling Indian crafts in 1923 and continued the business along with his wife, Sadie, until his death in 1968. The business stayed in the family until it was sold in 1972. Then in the mid-1980s, Skip Maisel, grandson of Maurice, reopened the store at the 510 Central Avenue location, where it continues today. The photograph below shows Maurice and Ethel at home, while the above photograph was taken just inside the front door of the store. Maurice and Ethel are on the left with two unidentified individuals, flanking a "wooden Indian" that sat in the store for many years. (Both, courtesy of Skip Maisel.)

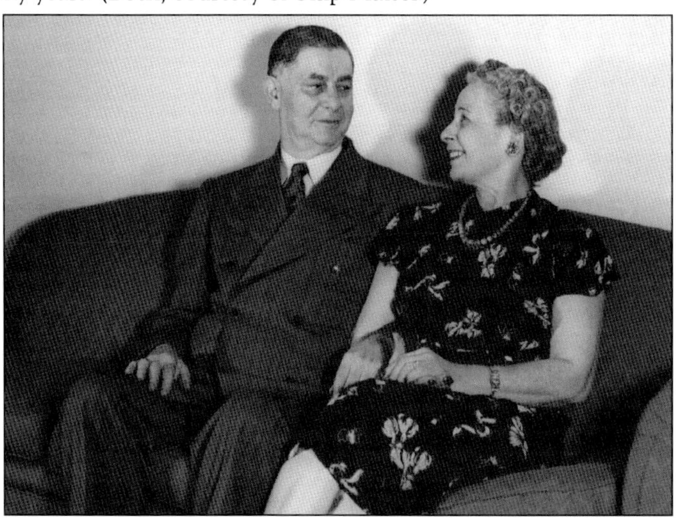

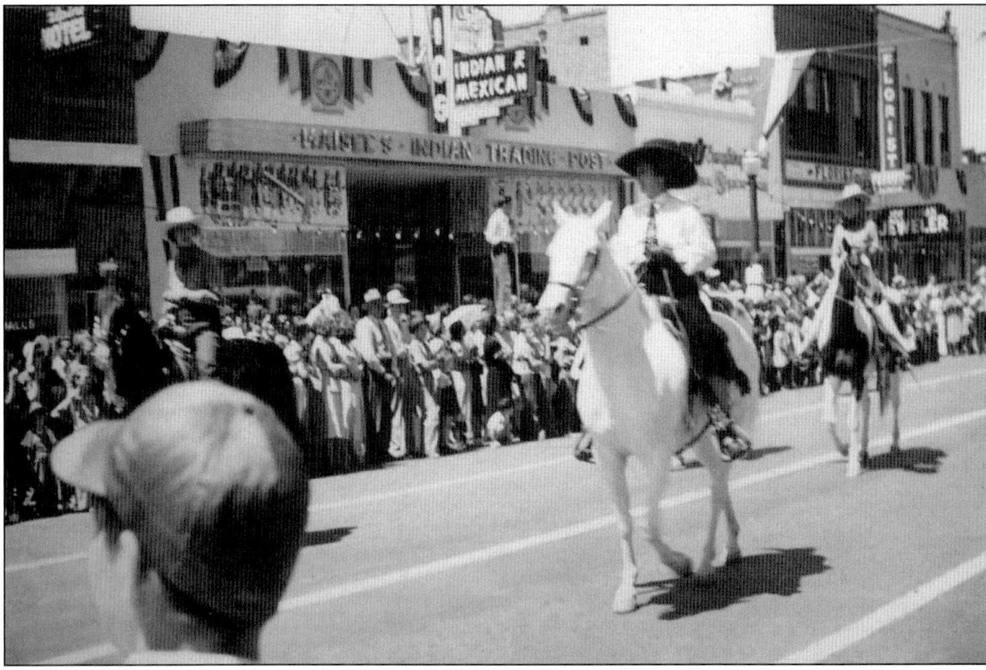

Maude Harris Dyer (1899–1998) rides by Maisel's on a grand white horse during what is possibly a Fourth of July parade sometime in the late 1930s. Clarence and Maude Dyer were longtime residents of Albuquerque who owned a ranch in Santa Fe County as well as cafés in Albuquerque. They were active in the Albuquerque Mounted Patrol. The picture below shows the terrazzo thunderbird at the store's entrance. There are silver dollars and pesos set into the design. (Above, courtesy of Gene Dyer; below, courtesy of Skip Maisel.)

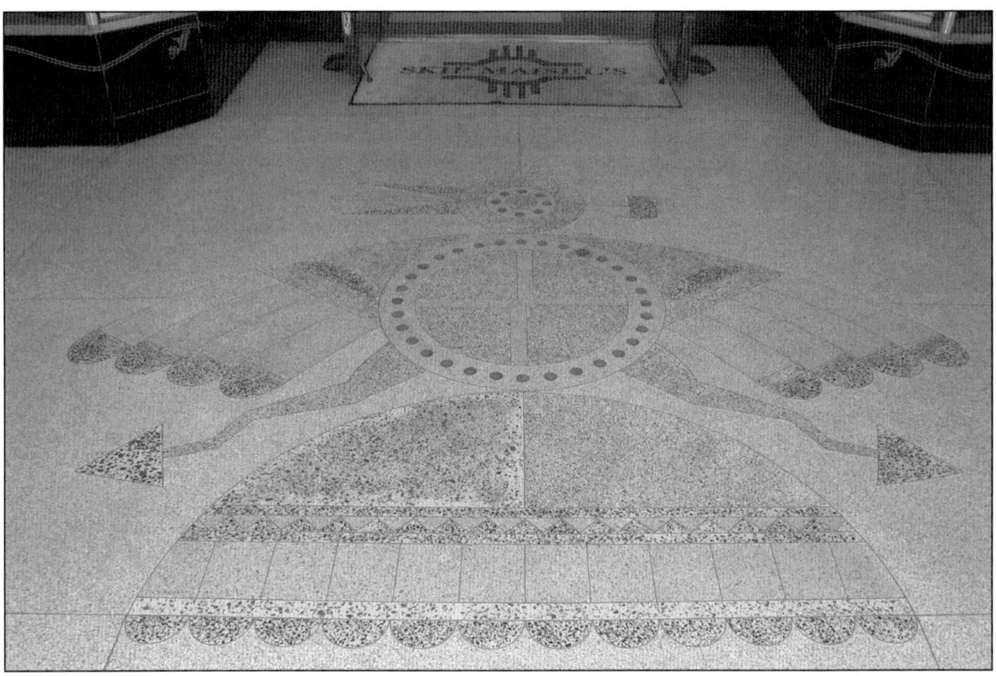

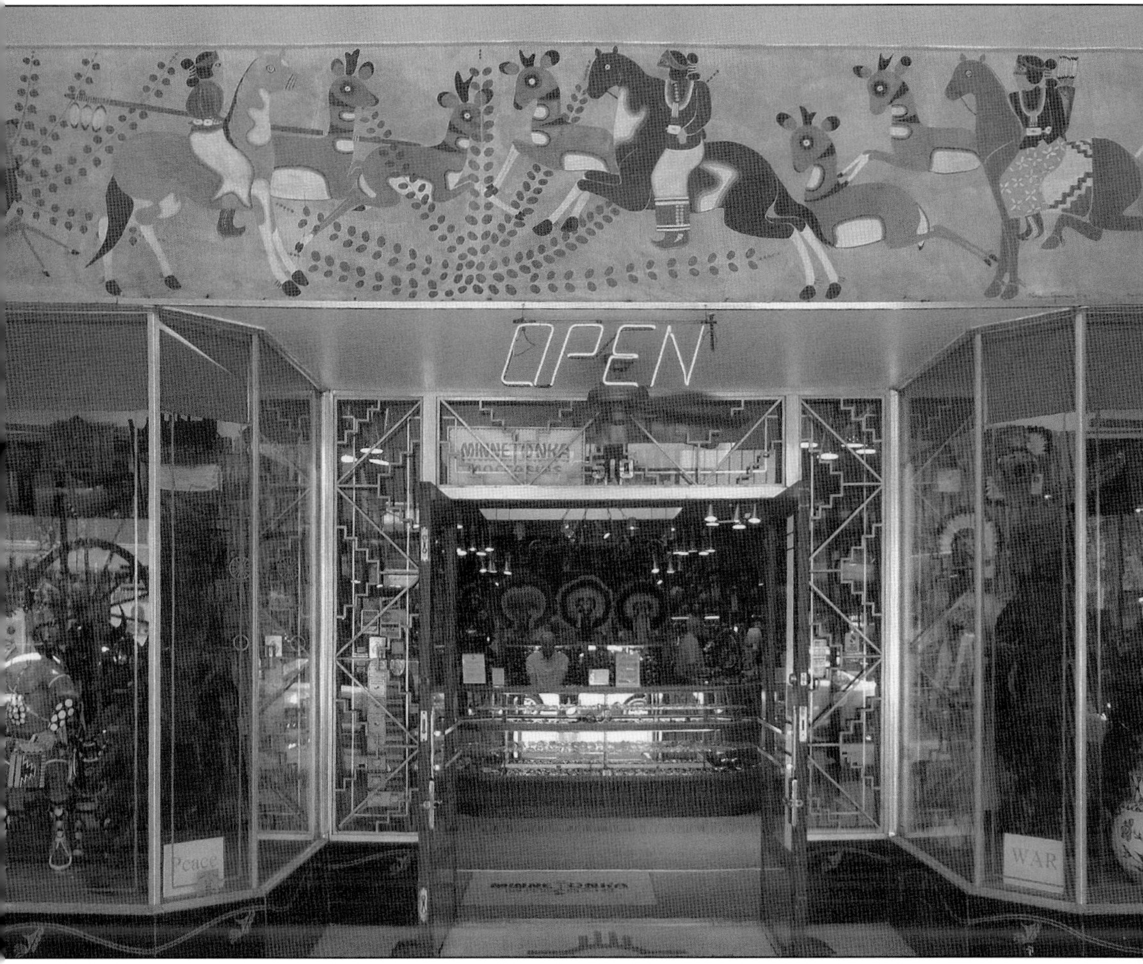

The entrance is modeled after a store that Maurice Maisel saw in Los Angeles; it is known that he provided a photograph of it, now lost, to architect Meem. Called Shaver's (or Schafer's), the building apparently had a curved Streamline Moderne front. However, Maisel preferred to have the expansive front display area rendered in an angular form. The 40 feet of murals fronting Maisel's are one of the few examples of Native American workmanship on a building of the time. They are pictured and described in total in chapter seven of this book. (Courtesy of Skip Maisel.)

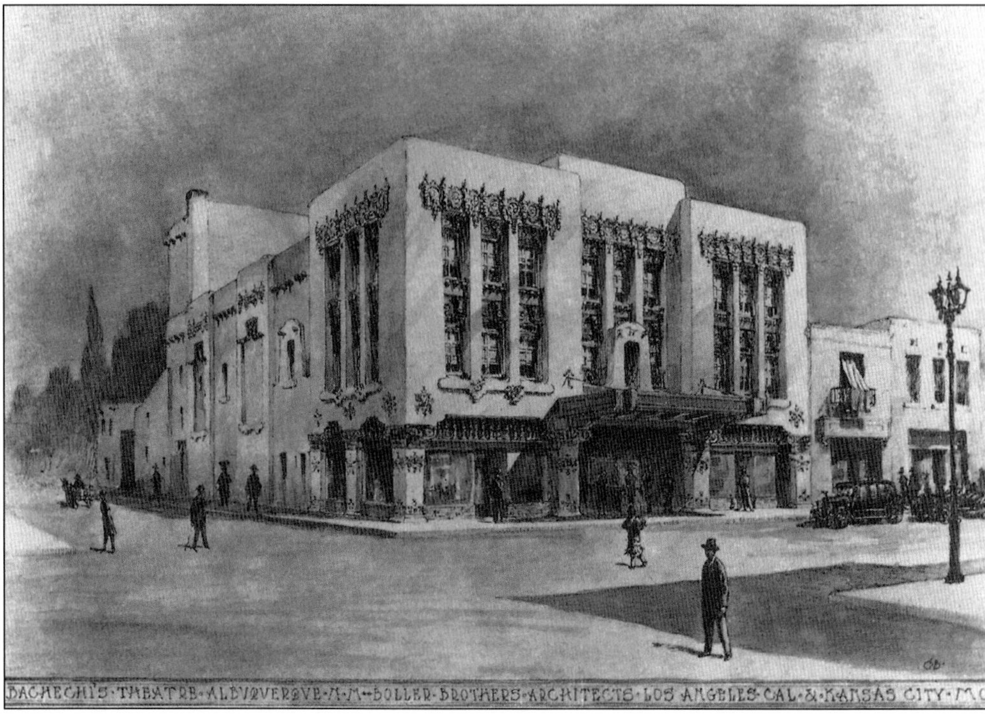
BACHECHI'S·THEATRE·ALBUQUERQUE·N.M.·BOLLER·BROTHERS·ARCHITECTS·LOS ANGELES·CAL·&·KANSAS CITY·MO

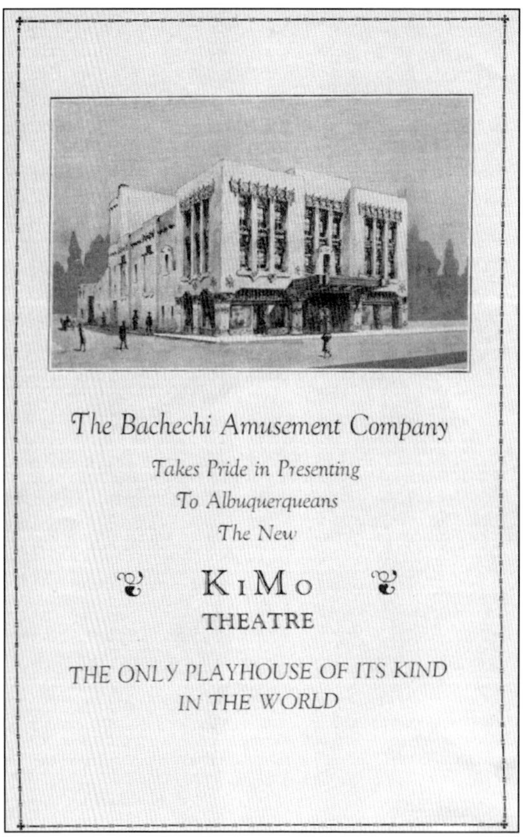
The Bachechi Amusement Company
Takes Pride in Presenting
To Albuquerqueans
The New
KiMo
THEATRE
THE ONLY PLAYHOUSE OF ITS KIND
IN THE WORLD

The Kimo Theater, at the northeast corner of Fifth Street and Central Avenue, was designed by Carl Boller. Boller Brothers architectural firm of Kansas City and Los Angeles designed many vaudeville theaters and movie palaces across the West. He was assisted by local architect/engineer George Williamson, who started his career with Trost & Trost. The Kimo is the realized vision of Italian immigrant Oreste Bachechi (1860–1928). For more information, see Arcadia Publishing's *Italians in Albuquerque*. Here is Boller's watercolor rendering of the building and the cover of the opening night program on September 19, 1927. Before undertaking the Kimo design, Bachechi sent Boller on a trip around the Southwest to take in the local culture and decorative motifs. While the building massing is a typical theater, the Deco ornamentation, especially the interior, is a wonder to behold. Fortunately the building has been totally restored to its original glory. (Both, courtesy of the UNM CSWR Brochure and Flyer Collection.)

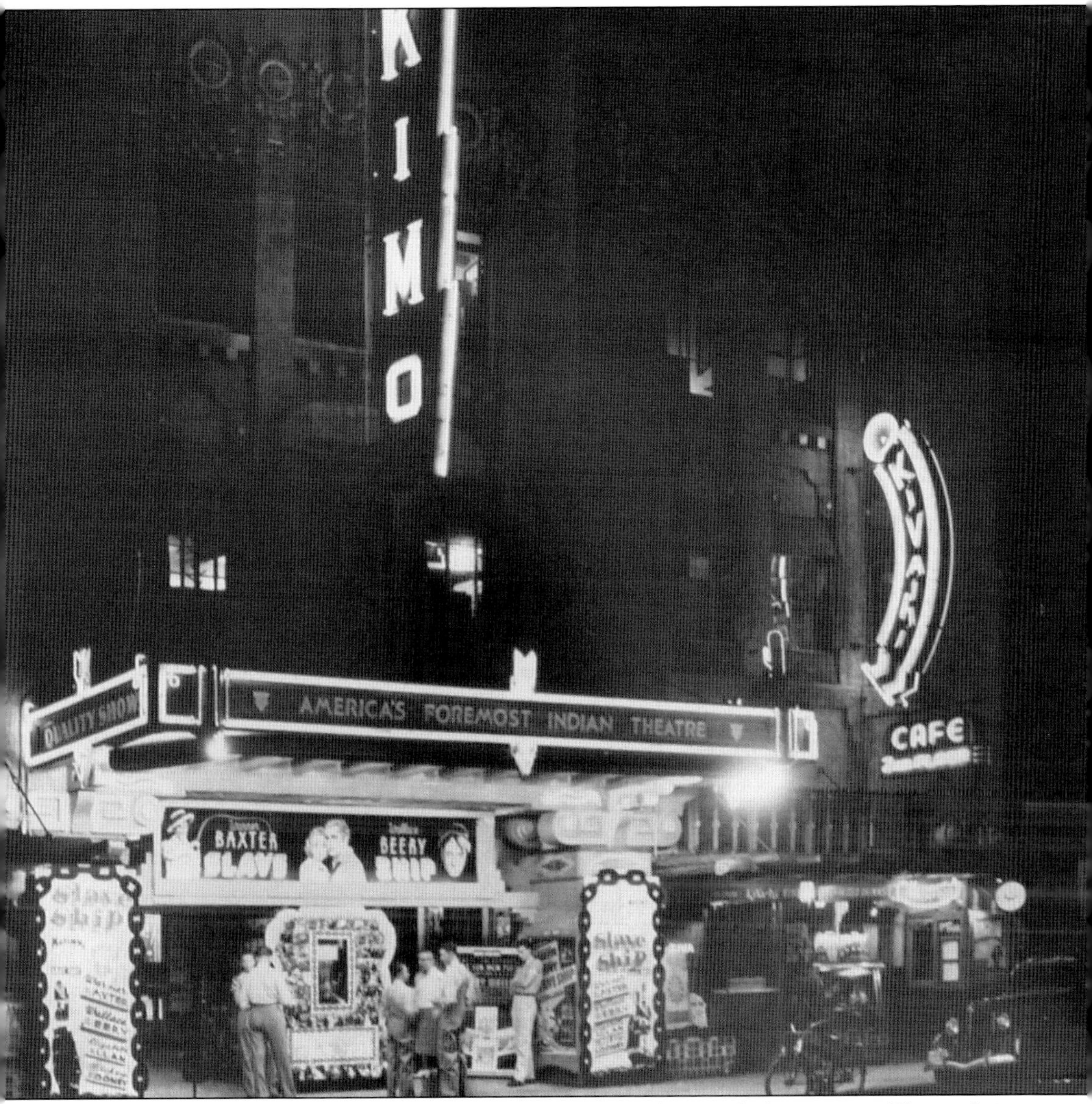

The Kimo's neon sign has recently been restored by the city, along with the marquee. This night view is from 1937, as identified by *Slave Ship* with Warner Baxter and Wallace Beery. Also prominent in the photograph is the adjoining Kiva Café. The ornamentation for the Kimo is nothing if not garish, with influences from regional Native American cultures, Spanish motifs, cowboys, and even a little Meso-American. Terra-cotta capitals with opposing frets, characteristic of Mayan buildings, are clearly visible here on either side of the marquee. Near the top of this picture are terra-cotta shield forms. Shields decorated with feathers and hangings were often carried by Indian participants in parades during the 1920s. Stepped cloud designs, highlighted by colored tile and tile bands, are also visible at the base of windows. (Courtesy of the Kimo Theater.)

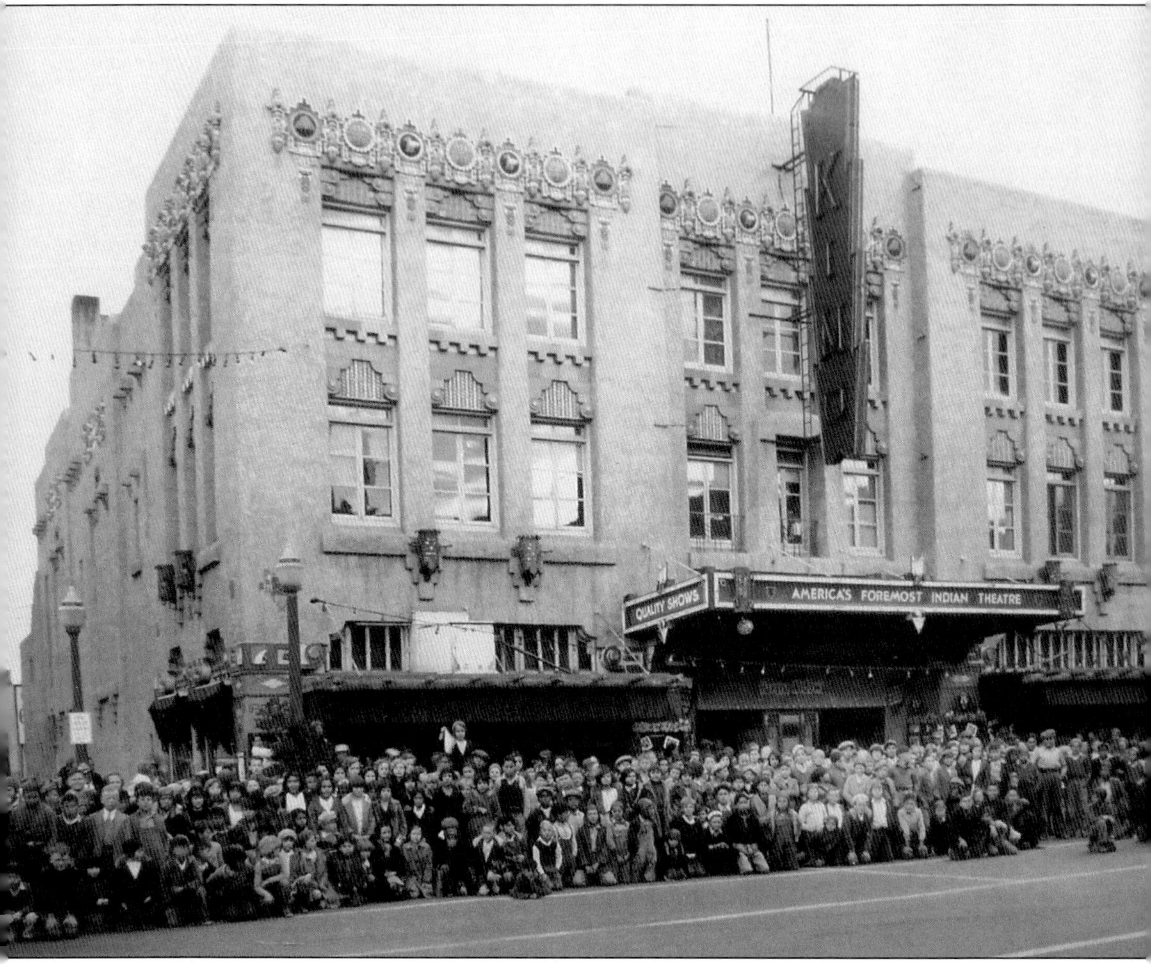

Here is a 1933 picture of the front of the Kimo with what looks to be every elementary school kid in Albuquerque. Why they are posed here is not known, although probably not to see the 1933 Joan Blondell comedy *Havana Widow* advertised on the marquee. The shields and window designs are well shown on this picture. The shield faces have alternating triangle, whirling log, and animal motifs. The hanging feathers and other hangings are reminiscent of the *faldoncito*, i.e. hanging designs found on Mexican baroque architecture. Metal lanterns with rather evil looking faces glare out below the first-story windows. Kimo, a combination of two Tiwa words, literally means "Mountain Lion," but is often referred to as meaning "King of its Kind." Isleta Pueblo governor Pablo Abeita won $50 for suggesting this name. (Courtesy of the Kimo Theater.)

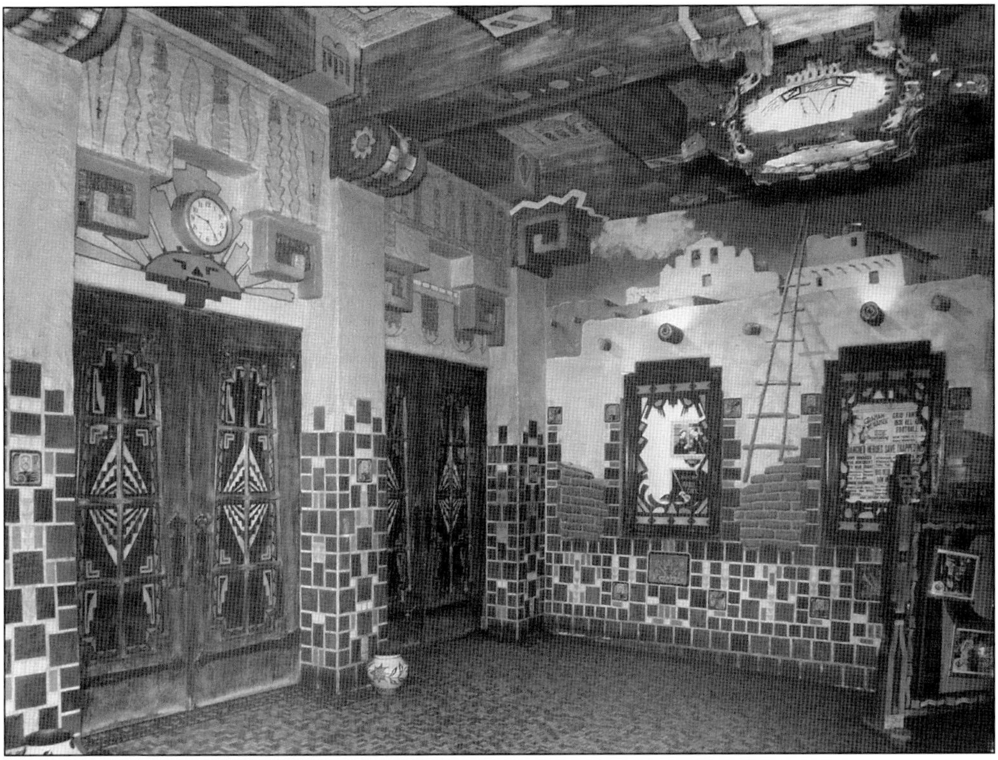

The 1936 Errol Flynn movie *Charge of the Light Brigade* had little to do with the actual event, but it provides a good starting point for entering the theater. The ticket taker stands at the ready and the arrows fronting the marquee point the way. Once past the ticket booth the wonder really begins. Native American symbolism is everywhere. Above each of the front doors is a *kachina* face, a sunburst, Mayan frets, and painted Pueblo-style wands. The hanging light fixture is said to represent a Native American funeral canoe. The Pueblo murals continue into the lobby, as do the carved and painted ceiling beams. The carved and painted doors have rug and pottery designs, and even the door handles are shaped like *kachina* figures. (Both, courtesy of the Kimo Theater.)

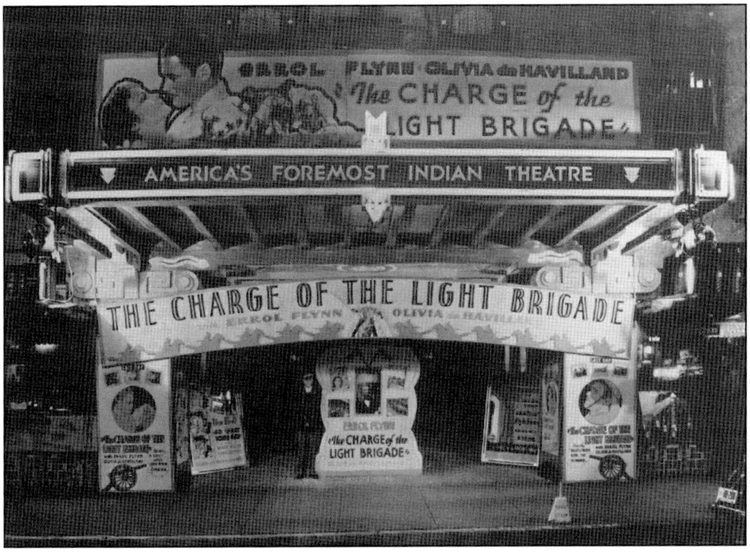

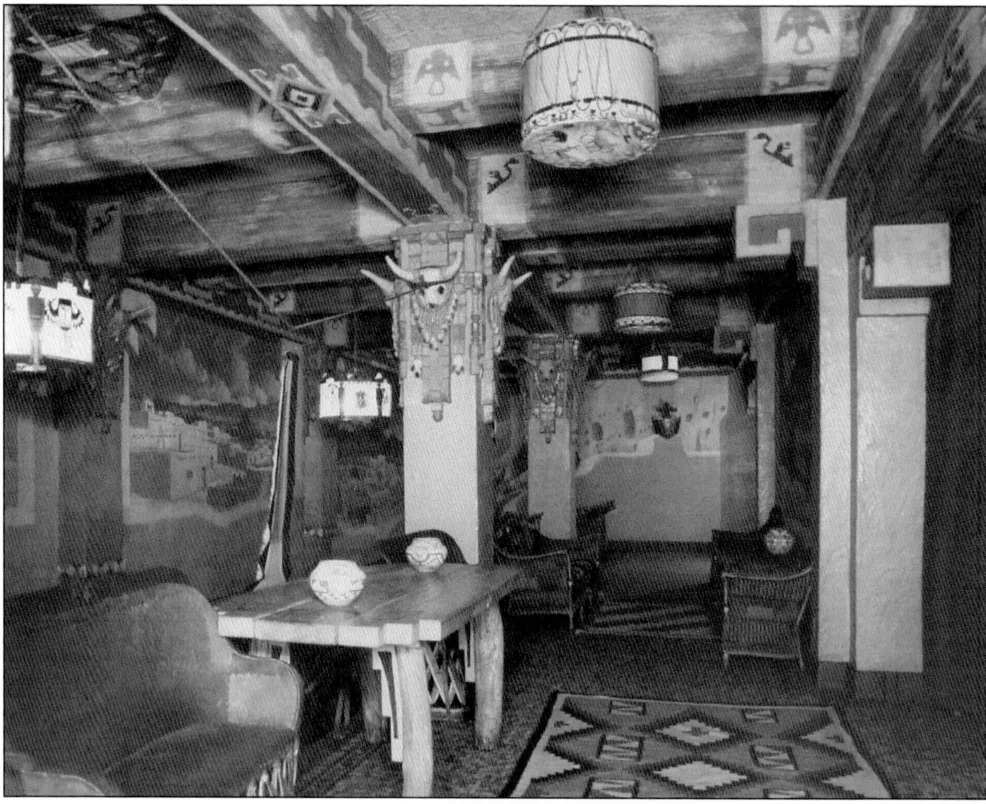

Pictured here is the lobby. In addition to architect Boller, designer Inez Barnes Westlake (1883–1943) also worked on the interior. She had previously assisted architects Trost & Trost on the Hotel Franciscan interiors pictured in the following chapter. The lobby and mezzanine have a typical theater layout, but the decoration at the Kimo is like no other. Above are drum-shaped ceiling fixtures as well as hanging lanterns with painted *kachinas* and masks. Rustic furniture and Navajo rugs accent the waiting area. Painted ceiling beams have animal figures and birds. Bird designs also adorn the metal staircase and balcony railing. A namesake mountain lion (Kimo) skin is visible hanging over the balcony in both of these photographs. (Both, courtesy of the Kimo Theater.)

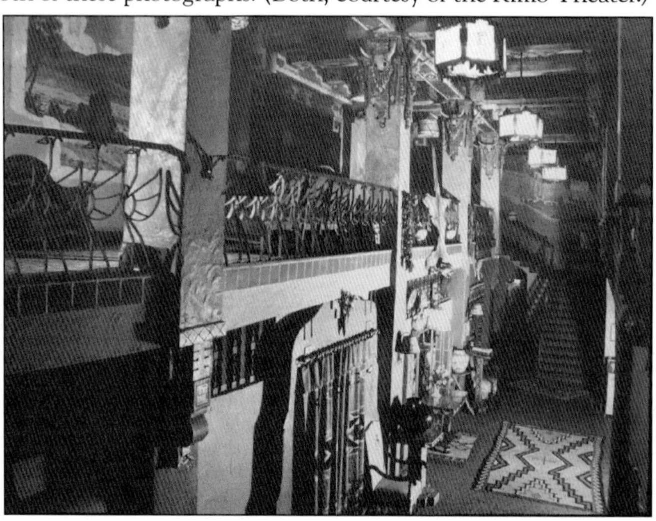

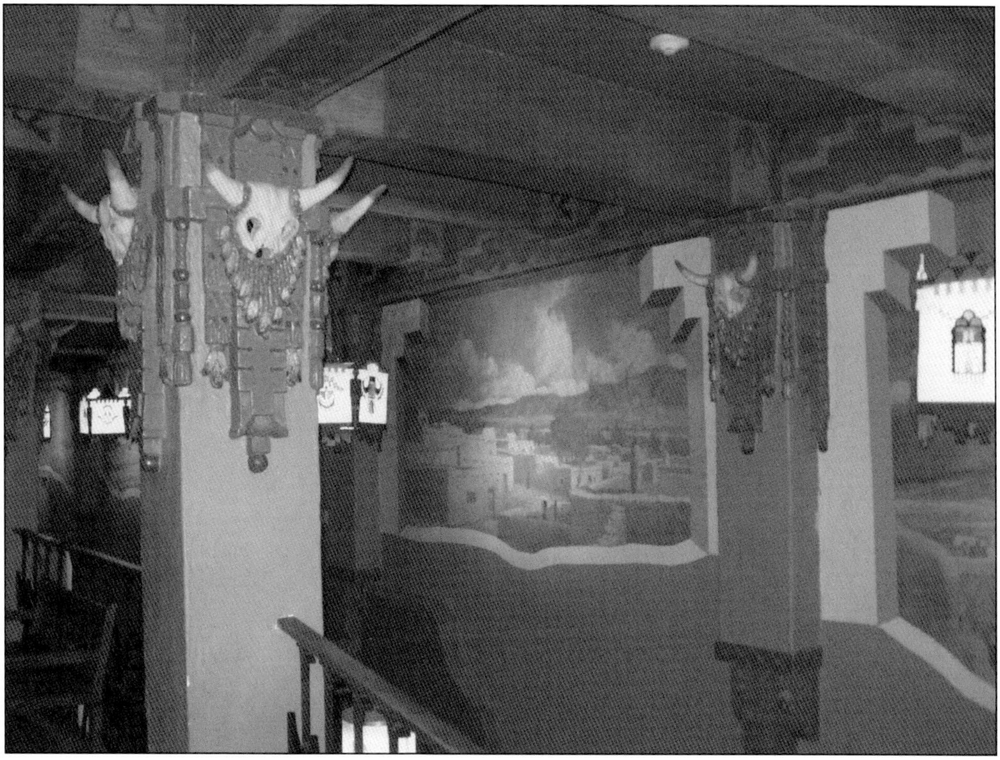

These photographs highlight the mezzanine murals painted by a German artist who moved to New Mexico in 1922 and settled in Albuquerque. Carl Von Hassler (1887–1969) was commissioned to portray the mythical *Seven Cities of Cibola*, which in fact are modeled after recognizable Pueblos, both historic and prehistoric. There are also several Southwest landscapes. White House ruin in Canyon de Chelly is at the top of the east stairs, while various Rio Grande and Hopi Pueblos grace the mezzanine. Von Hassler apparently accompanied Bolling on the preparatory tour of the Southwest and then spent months painting the murals. It is also said that Bachechi instructed him on their composition. The plaster cow skulls add another touch of the Southwest, if there was any confusion about where one is. (Both, courtesy of the Kimo Theater.)

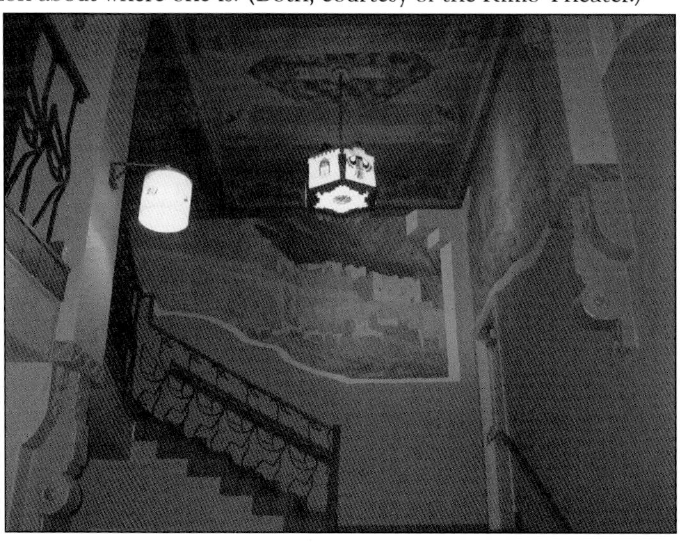

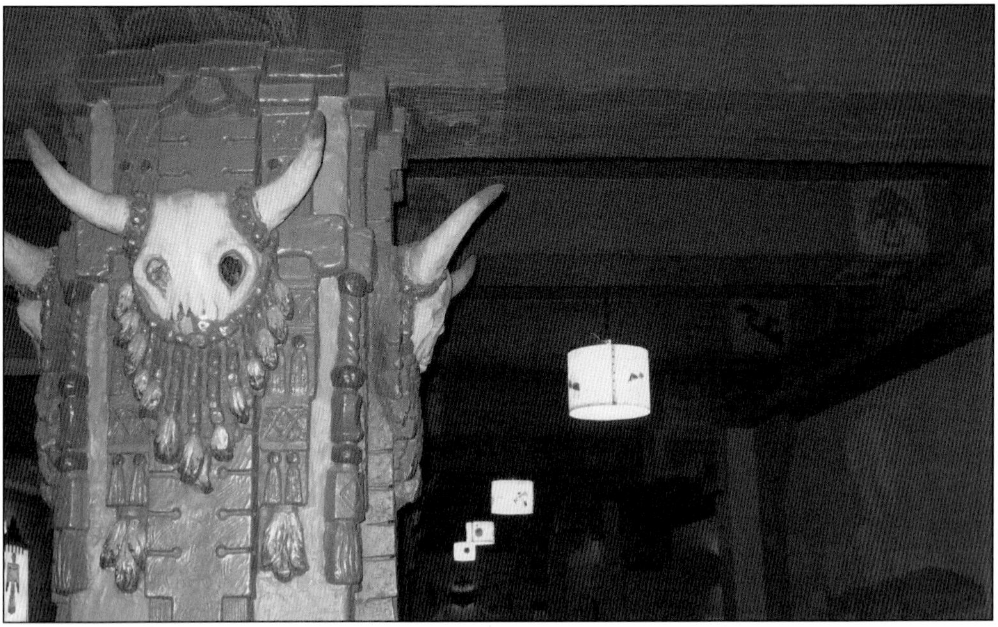

The cow skulls of cast plaster painted with high gloss enamel have lighted red eyes. These skulls, with knotted cord and feather hangings, are on all four sides of the capitals supporting the mezzanine, between shields lining the main auditorium, and arching above the stage. Paintings of Navajo *Yei* (God) figures also adorn the auditorium walls. The heads of two such figures are visible on the photograph below. (Both, courtesy of the Kimo Theater.)

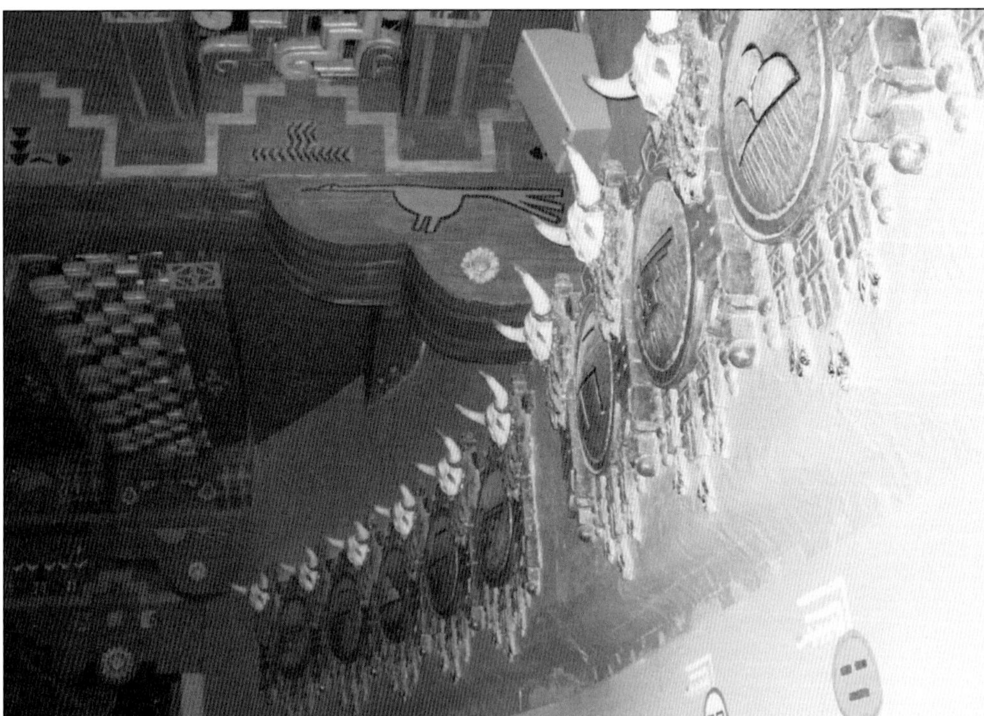

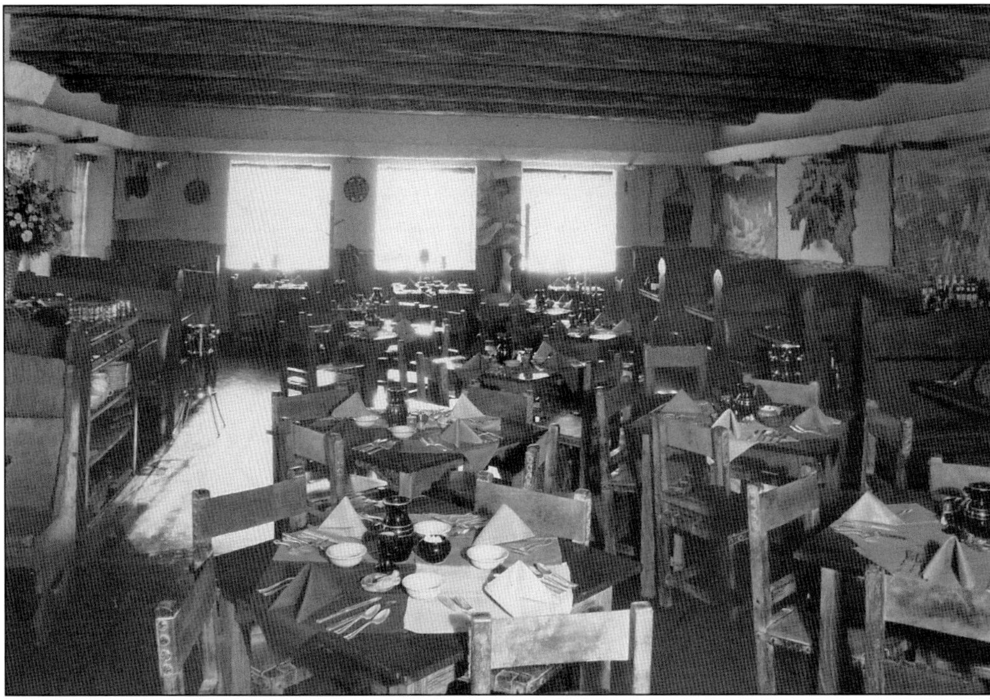

A restaurant and a gift shop were located in spaces adjacent to the theater entry. Here is a picture of the lunch counter and restaurant seating room (the Kiva Café) east of the main entrance. There are painted tepee awnings over some of the side tables, and Pueblo pots above the counter area. There also appear to be Von Hassler paintings on the walls as well as a painted cowhide. (Both, courtesy of the Kimo Theater.)

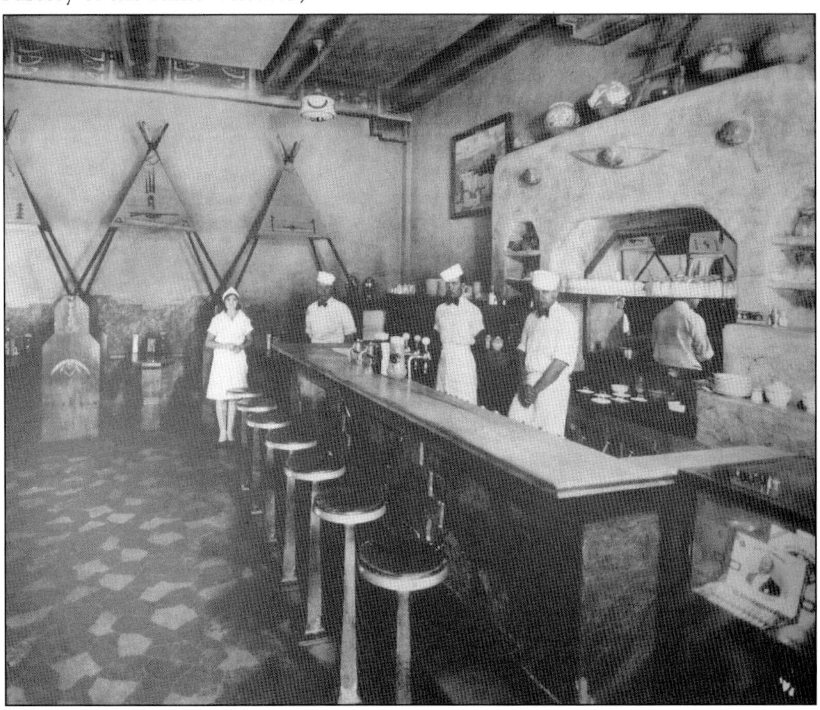

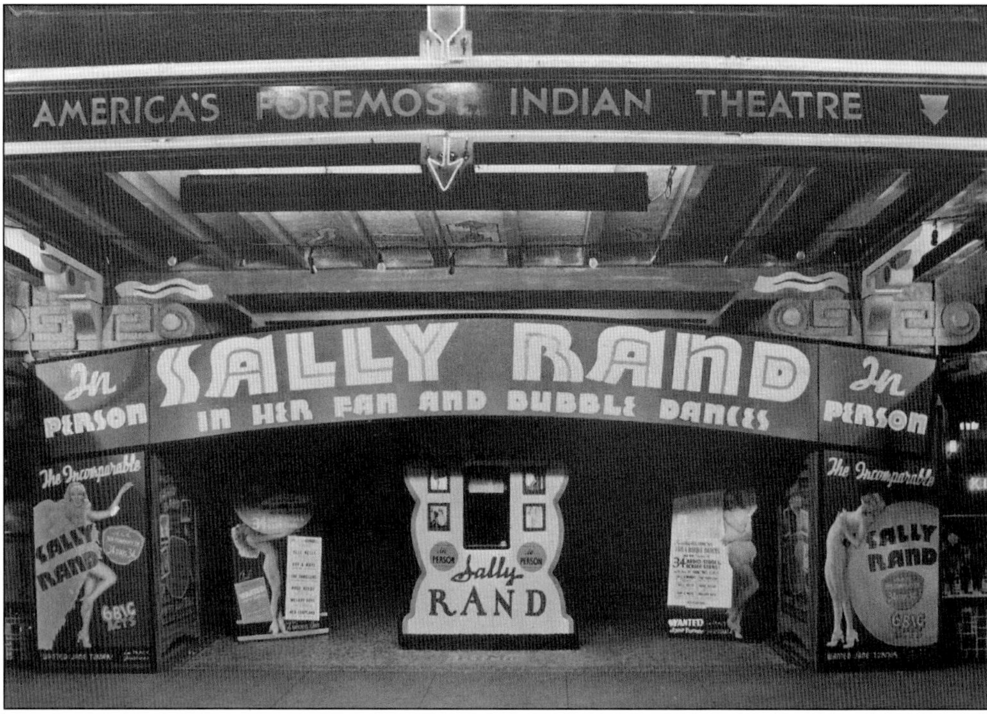

The Kimo was host to many of the popular acts of the day as well as major movies. Vivian Vance, who gained fame as Lucille Ball's sidekick in the *I Love Lucy* series, performed at the Kimo. The theater also hosted such stars as Sally Rand, Gloria Swanson, Tom Mix, and Ginger Rogers. When the theater was packed, the balcony—which spans the east to west walls without support and was designed to give and sway—would drop four to eight inches in the middle. The classic film *In Old Chicago* with Alice Faye and Tyrone Power is from 1937, while the Sally Rand fan and bubble dance looks to be from the late 1930s. (Both, courtesy of the Kimo Theater.)

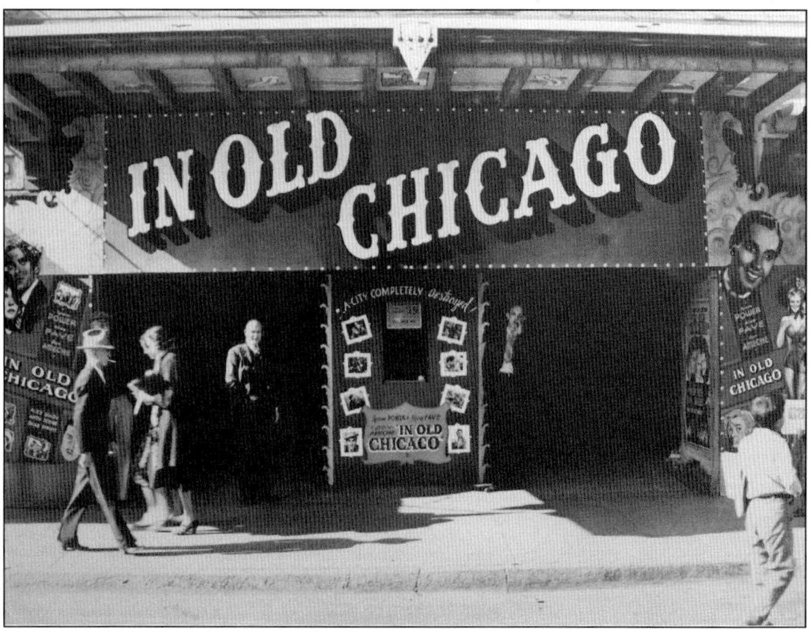

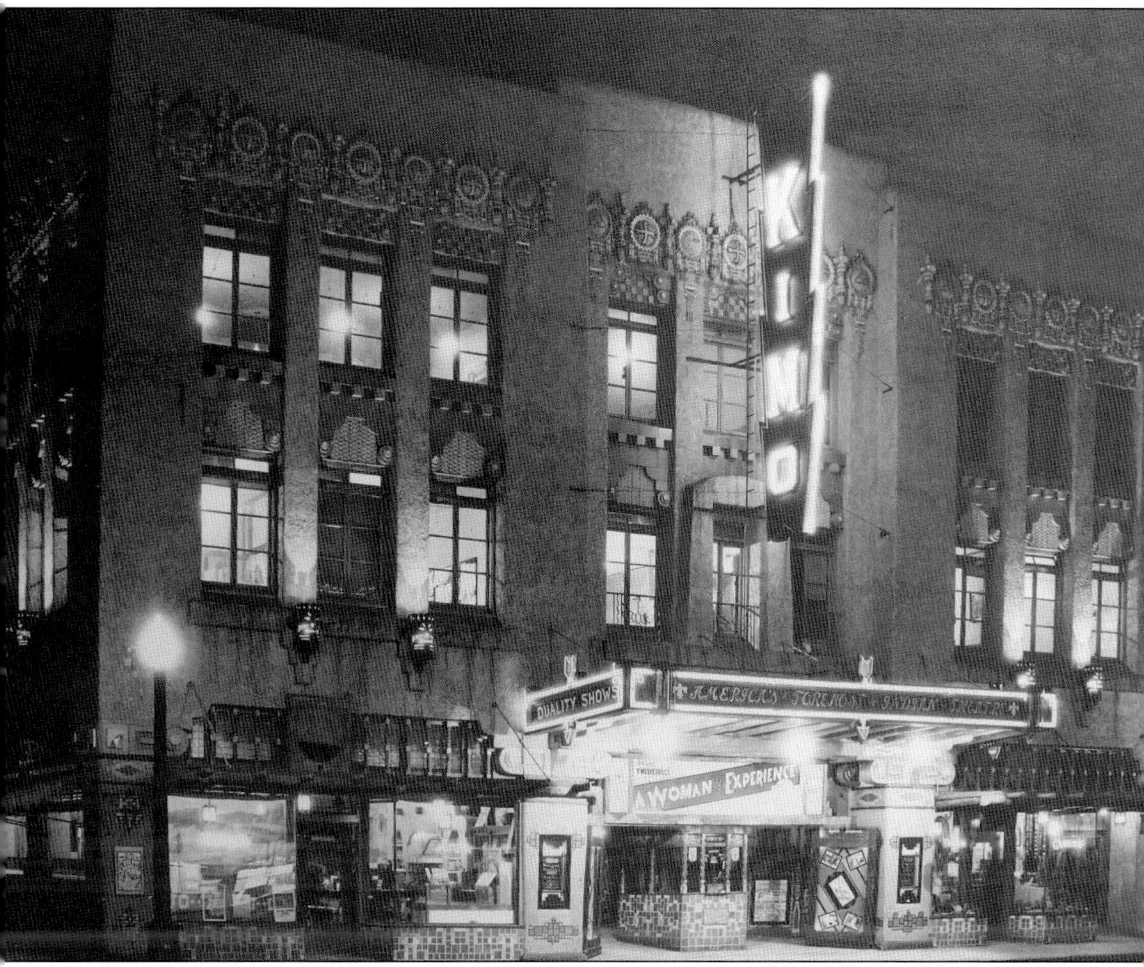

The theater, which cost $150,000, was completed in less than a year. Fortunately Oreste Bachechi lived to see it completed, as he died the year following his monument's opening. An elaborate Wurlitzer pipe organ that accompanied the silent films of the day was an extra $18,000. The overview of the Kimo closes with this night shot from 1931. The marquee shows that the current film was *A Woman of Experience*, starring Helen Twelvetrees and William Bakewell. (Courtesy of the Kimo Theater.)

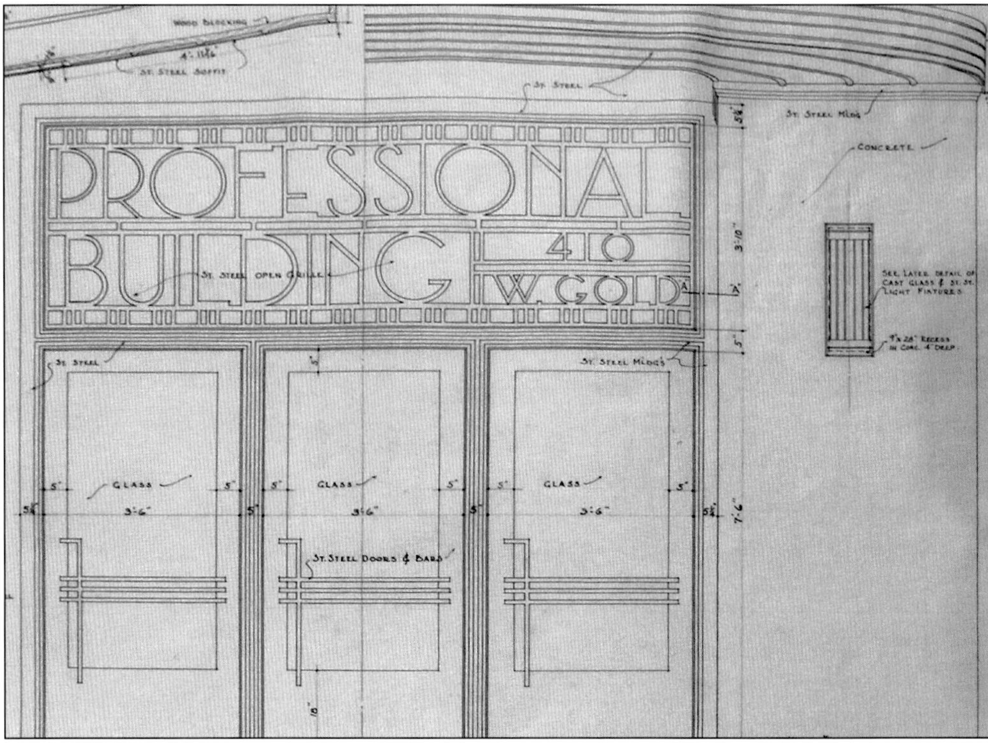

In 1937, John Gaw Meem was commissioned by Albert G. Simms, a local banker and politician, to design a 10-story office building at 410 West Gold Avenue. For this project, Meem put his typical revival architecture aside and designed a full on Art Deco skyscraper. Here, the details of the entry and elevator lobby are shown. Had it been constructed, it would have been the first real skyscraper in Albuquerque and certainly the city's most "modern" building. The building would have cost about $650,000, which was apparently too much at the time for Simms, although the land was acquired and the design brought to the stage of finished specifications. There is a rumor that Simms's wife did not like the design. (Both, courtesy of the UNM CSWR John Gaw Meem Archive.)

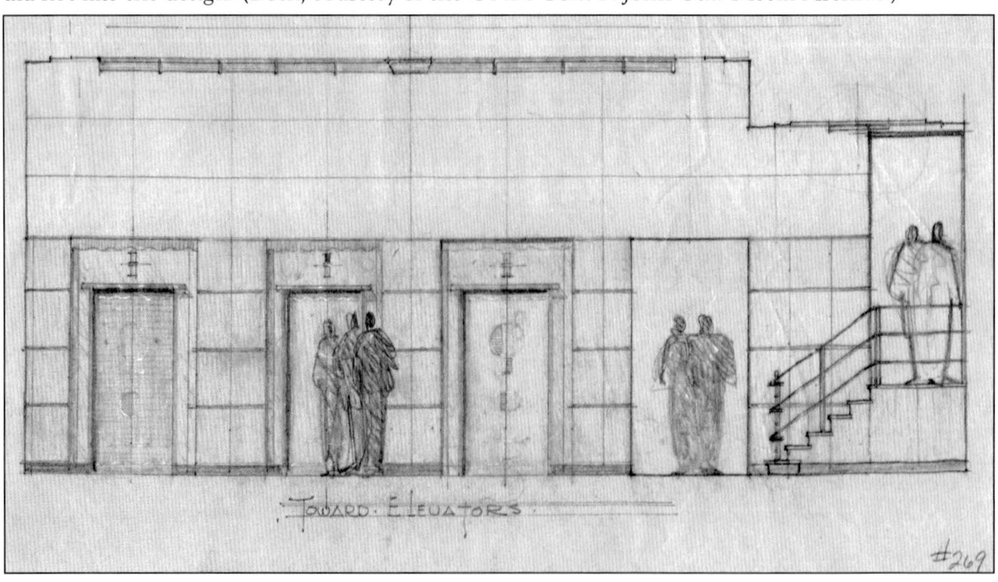

In 1954, on the same site as the 1937 project, the Simms Building was constructed. At the time, the 13-story International-style structure was the tallest building in the state. The architect was the local firm of Flatow, Moore, Bryan, and Fairburn. The Simms Building was listed in the National Register of Historic Places in 1998. It is seen here contrasted with Wright's Trading Post, a make-believe Indian Pueblo across the street along with a sketch of the building originally designed for the site. (Right, courtesy of the UNM CSWR John Gaw Meem Archive; below, courtesy of Nancy Tucker.)

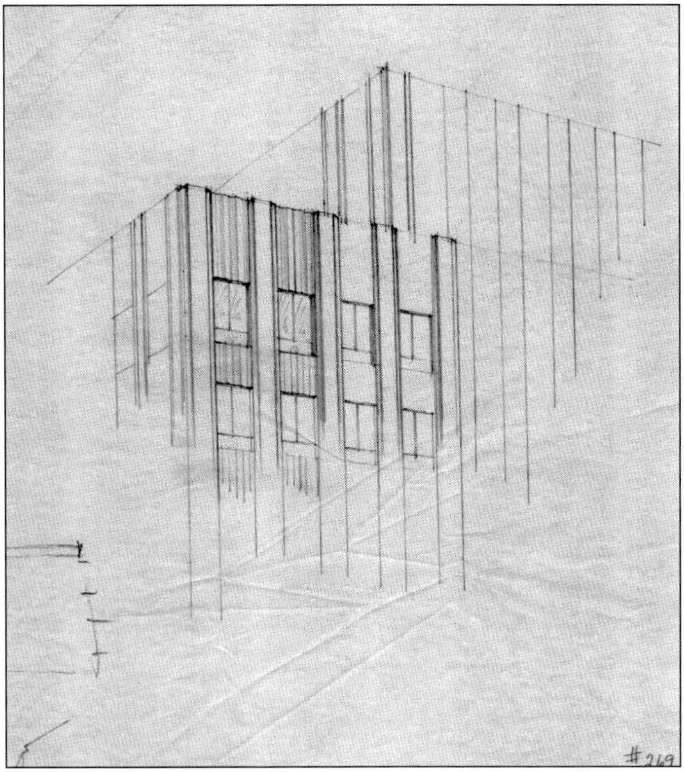

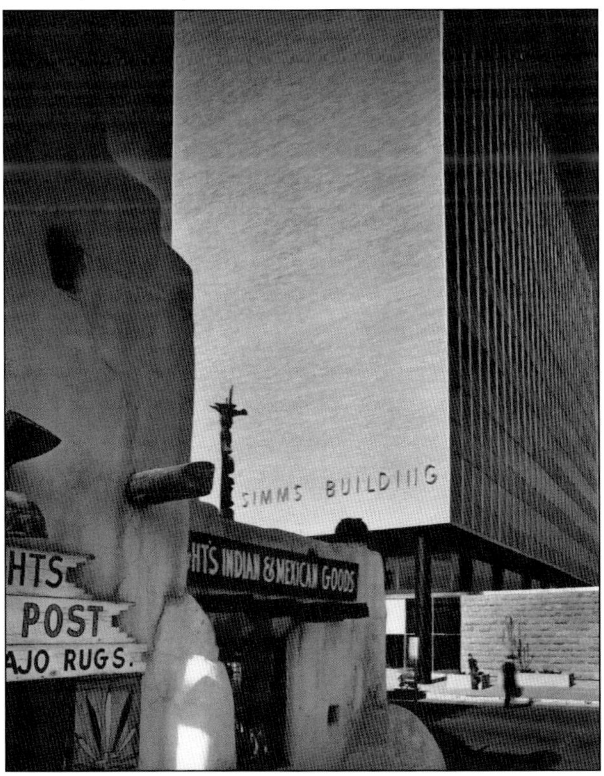

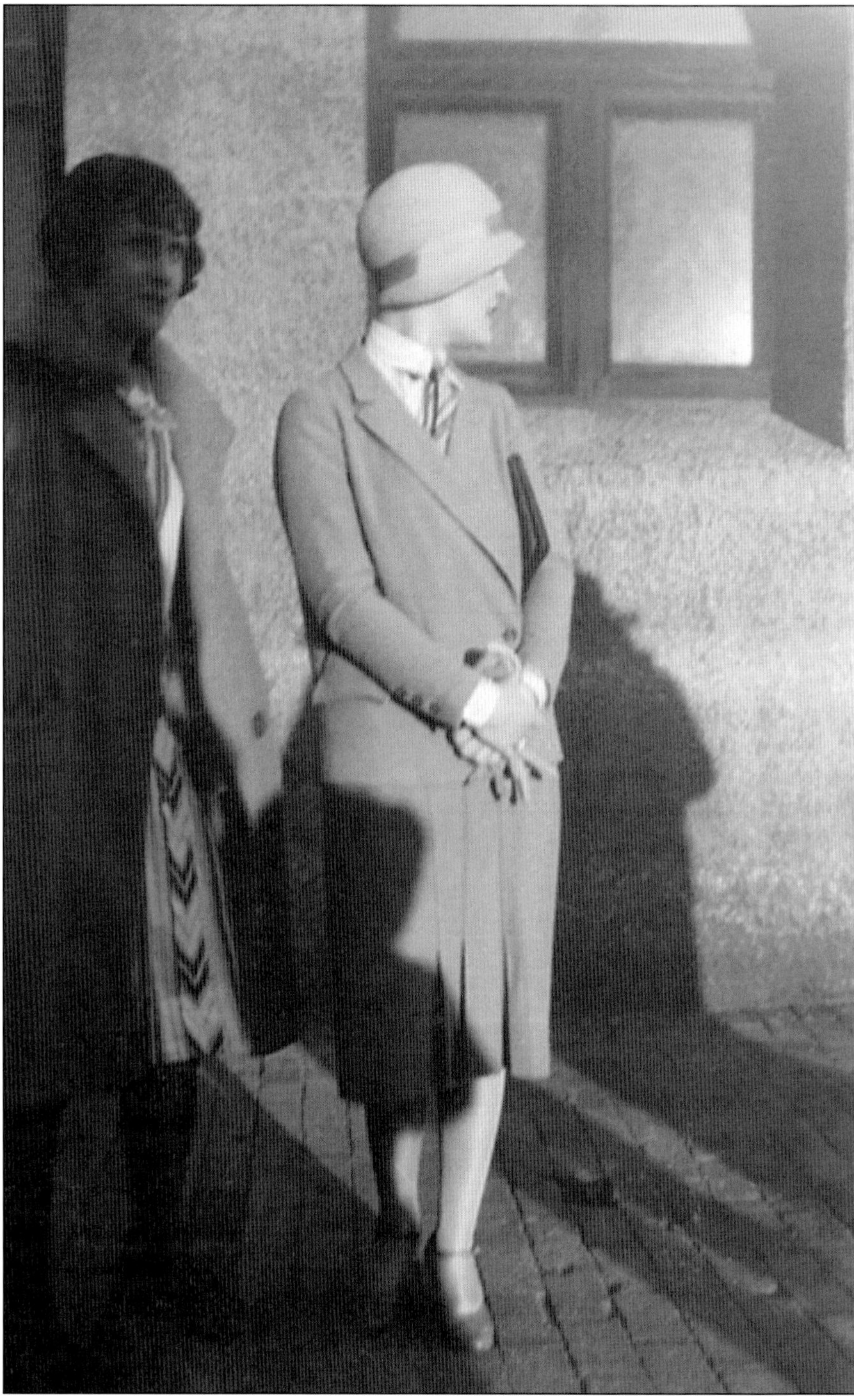

This chapter ends with Laura La Plante (1904–1996) on the train station platform by the Alvarado Hotel in 1926; the hat is certainly Deco. At this time she was the most popular star of Universal Pictures. Only in her mid-20s when the talkies arrived, La Plante proved to be a quite natural and appealing presence but the huge wave of new stars in those years overshadowed her. She made her last appearances for Universal in 1930. (Courtesy of the Albuquerque Museum.)

Five

HOTELS

Four hotels, each in a distinctive architectural style, are presented in this chapter. The first is the Mission Revival–style Alvarado (1901), a railroad hotel. The history of this most iconic of Harvey Houses has been covered in a number of other books. The concentration here is principally on its architectural features. A careful look shows more Spanish-Pueblo influence than is usually attributed to the structure. The Spanish-Pueblo-Mayan inspired Franciscan Hotel (1923), demolished shortly after the Alvarado, was once a solid anchor at the west end of the downtown business district on Route 66, serving train, air and automotive travelers. The Territorial-style Hilton Hotel (1939), principally a business hotel in the middle of downtown, has fortunately been beautifully restored, at least the first two floors. The lobby has a decidedly Mission feel, with Western murals, along with southwestern details. Last is the Shaffer Hotel in the small town of Mountainair south of Albuquerque. Usually it is referred to as Pueblo Deco, but if there was ever a building to be called "Coyote Deco," this is it! The basic building is a concrete box. However, the ornamentation is a vernacular tour de force. Fortunately, this hotel has been preserved in nearly original condition, right down to the handmade chairs in the dining room and lobby.

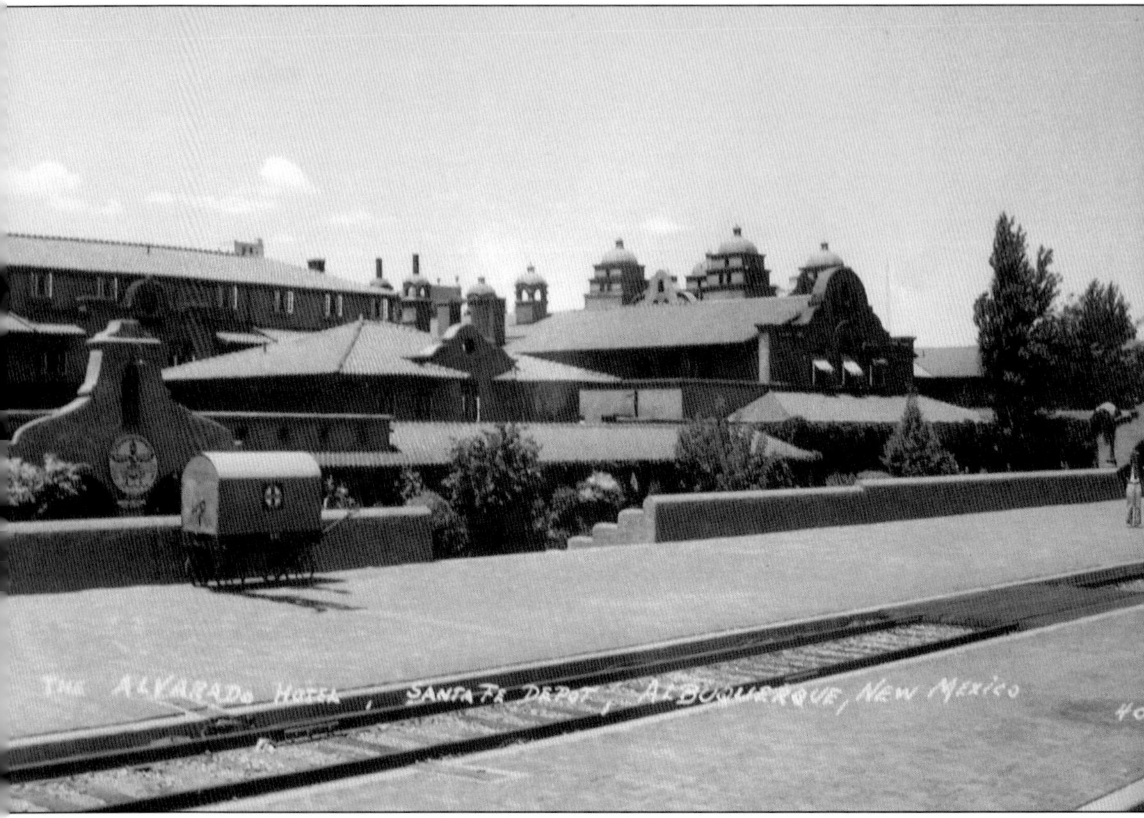
THE ALVARADO HOTEL, SANTA FE DEPOT, ALBUQUERQUE, NEW MEXICO
40

The 1902 Alvarado Hotel and the Santa Fe Railway station next to it were designed by Charles Whittlesey, a protégé of Louis Sullivan, who went out on his own and moved from Chicago to Albuquerque to work on Santa Fe projects. The complex of buildings also included office space and employee housing, making Albuquerque the administrative center for the Santa Fe/Fred Harvey companies' southwestern operations. The Alvarado complex is directly inspired by California Mission architecture. There are specific architectural references that relate to the tripartite towers from the Santa Barbara Mission and to other California missions. This is a form that probably also appeared occasionally in New Mexico but was essentially lost by the 19th century. In addition, there are numerous bell arches common to both California and New Mexico missions. Some seem to derive from portions of the bell arches at the San Gabriel Mission. (Courtesy of Nancy Tucker.)

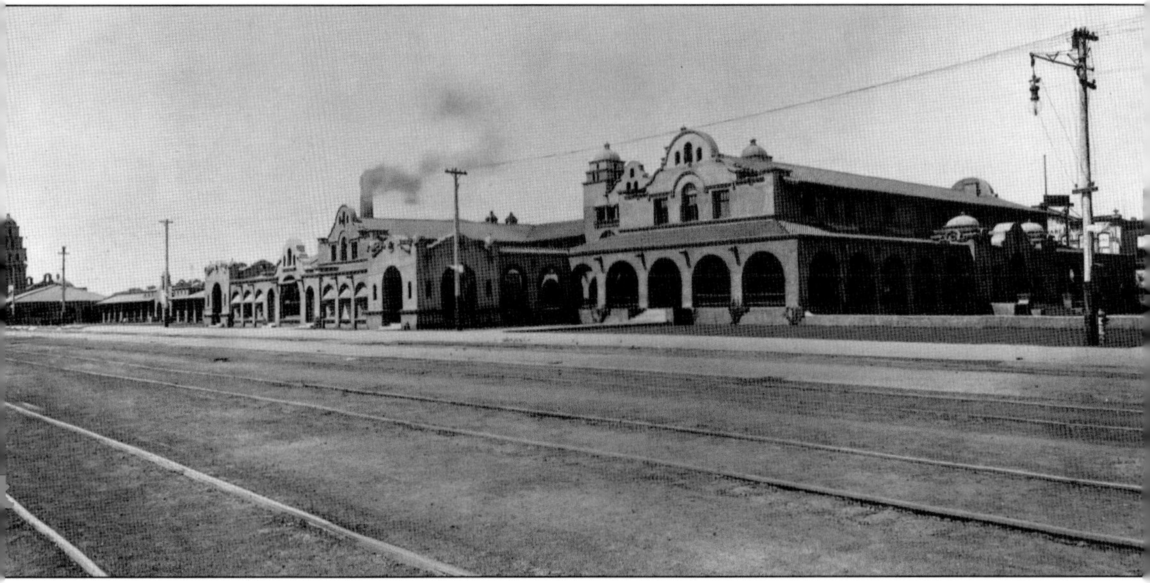

The Alvarado includes details from the San Diego Mission as well as entry arches and colonnades derived from the San Luis Rey Mission. The facades, bell arches, entrances, and parapets for various buildings of this complex give the impression that one is looking at a collection of mission churches, rather than a single church, with associated structures such as a *convento*. The rough stucco walls, a trademark of Santa Fe Railroad architecture, contrast with the typically smooth adobe walls of early New Mexico structures. But why was it Mission and not Pueblo style? This seems clearly to be an effort to convey a more "restful" and "peaceful" image associated with the California missions in late-19th-century preservation and promotional literature, rather than the "rough" and "primitive" Pueblos. On the Santa Fe and at Fred Harvey's the traveler could have both worlds, in comfort. (Courtesy of Nancy Tucker.)

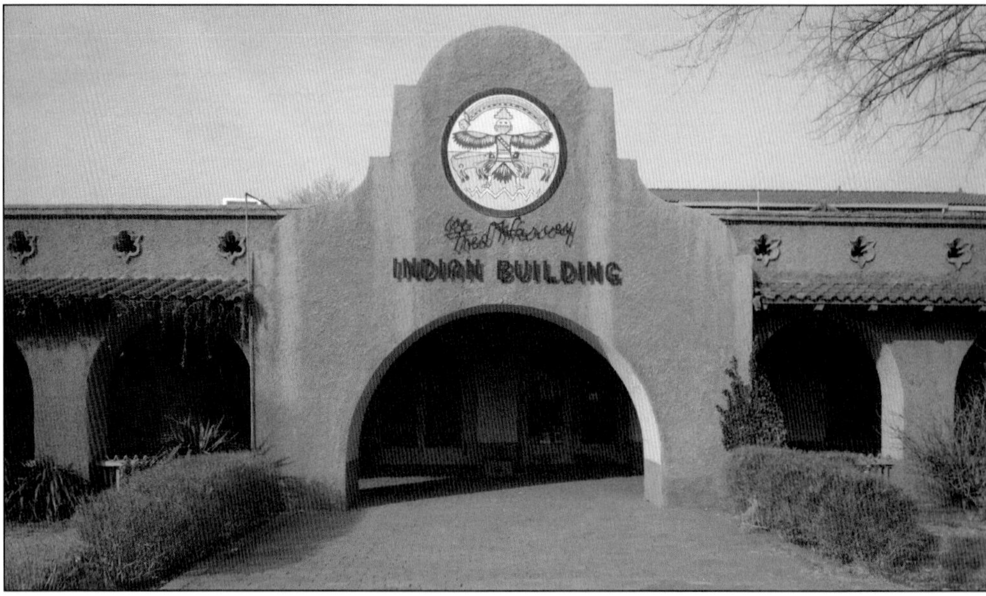

Pictured here are the east and west entrances of the Indian Building, a part of the hotel complex that contained Harvey's fabulous collection of Native American arts and crafts. The shop functioned as both museum display and sales emporium; a significant portion of the collection is now housed at the Heard Museum in Phoenix, Arizona. The simplified arches of the Alvarado complex are more suggestive of the Isleta *convento* (see page 18) than they are of California Mission colonnades and entrances. However, it seems most unlikely that Isleta would have been a model as all evidence of the Isleta colonnade was gone long before 1900. California Mission arches nearly always have suggestion of a capital at the top of a column supporting an arch. The star-shaped openings are reminiscent of the large star window above the entrance of San Carlos (Carmel) Mission. (Both, courtesy of the UNM CSWR Fred Harvey Collection.)

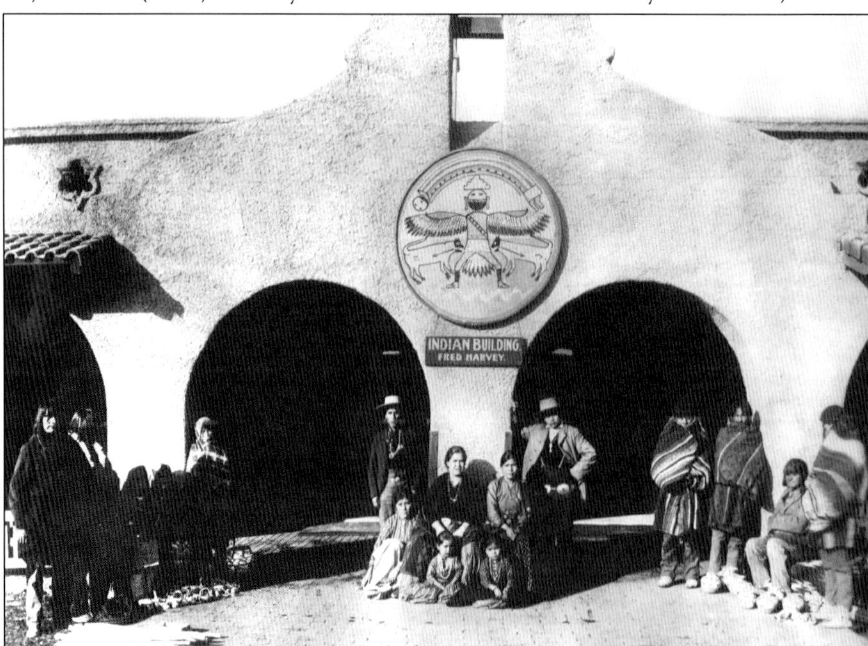

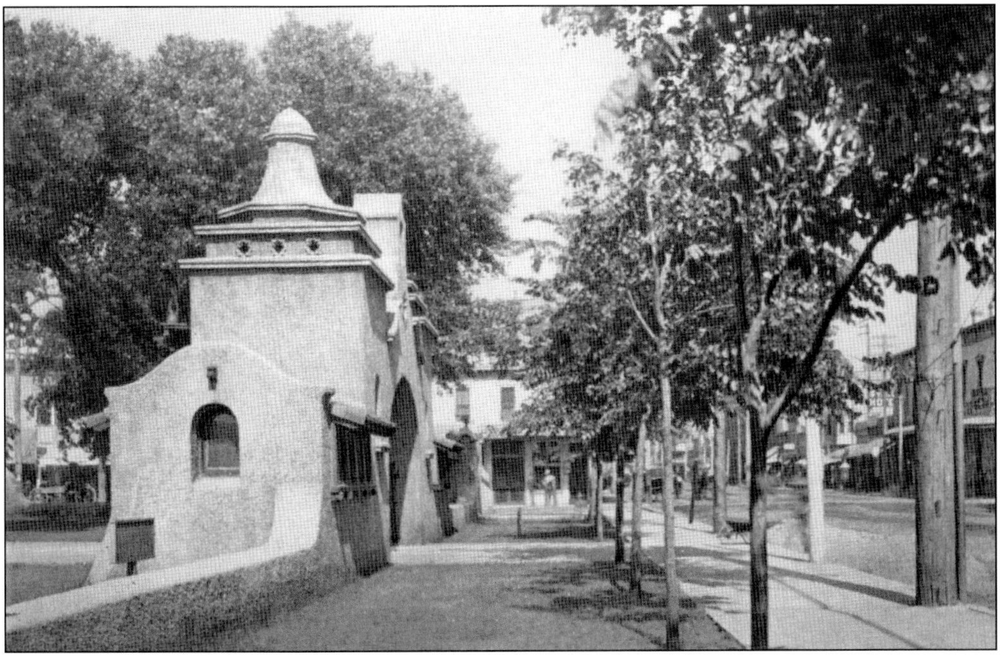

The entrances to the Alvarado complex were designed to evoke the serenity of a mission garden. Passengers exiting trains and persons entering the buildings from First Street passed though arches into walled gardens or arched colonnades that opened onto gardens. And looking from the dining room or a hotel room into a garden was undoubtedly soothing, given the constant rail activity and heat of summer before air-conditioning. (Both, courtesy of Nancy Tucker.)

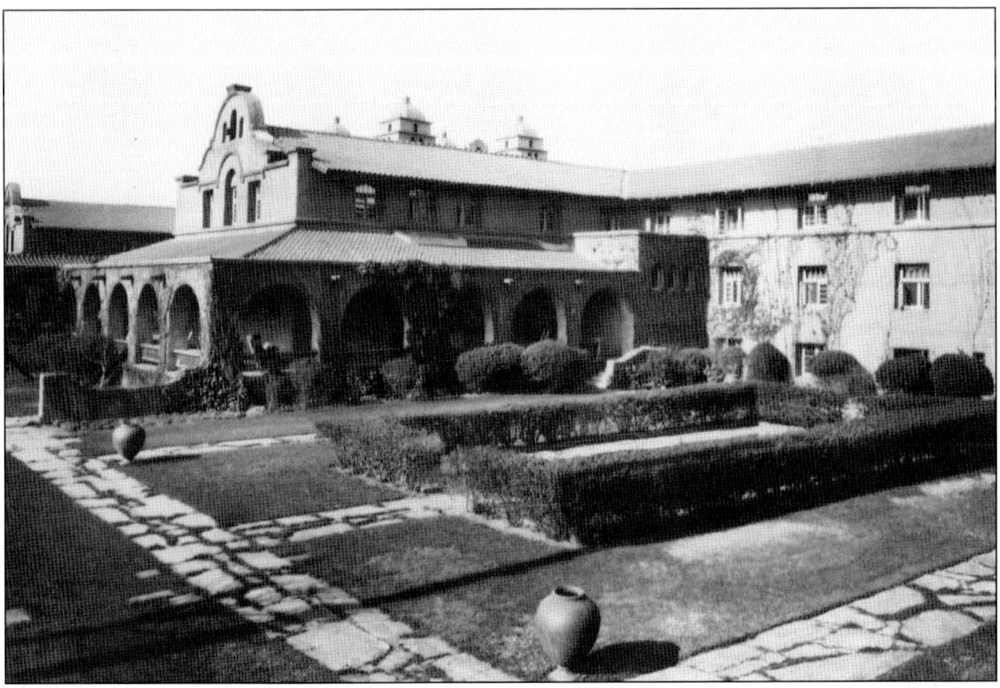

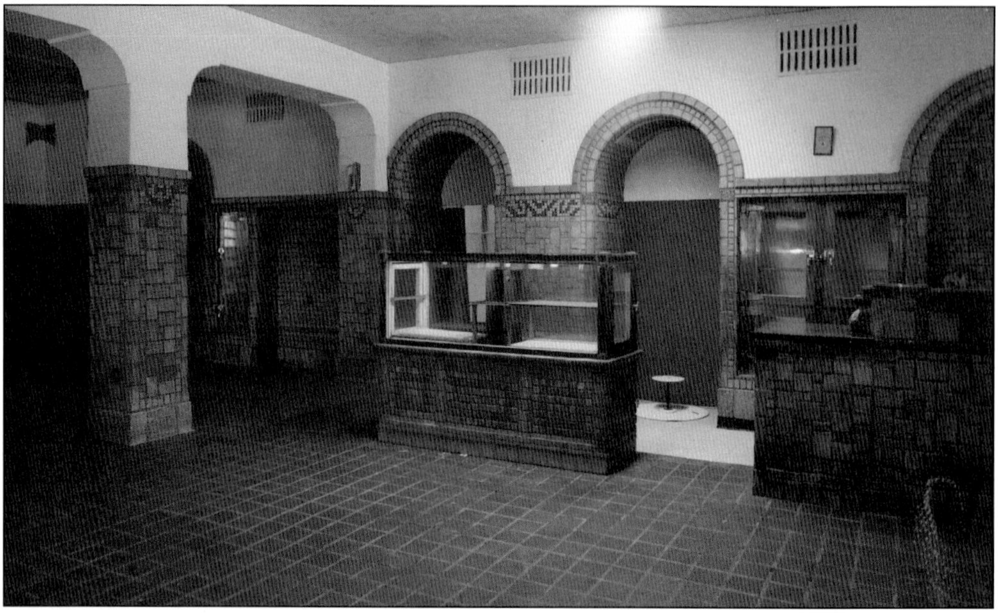

Alvarado interiors were a varied combination of southwestern objets d'art and Mission design plasterwork. Note the light-fixture mounts flanking the fireplace, along with wood trim and ceilings, as some are stenciled with Indian designs. Floors were either wooden planking or tile. Tile wainscoting and door surrounds were also common, often with rug or basketry designs. Often the tile work has a decidedly Arts and Crafts movement character. Architect Mary Colter (1869–1958) was responsible for many of the Fred Harvey interiors. (Both, courtesy of the National Archives, Historic American Building Survey.)

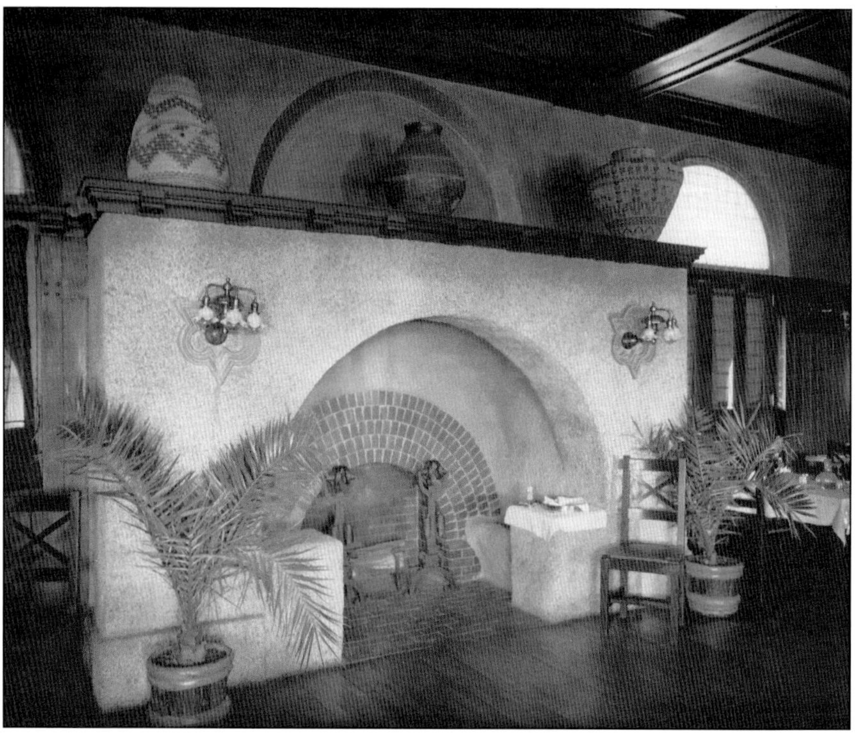

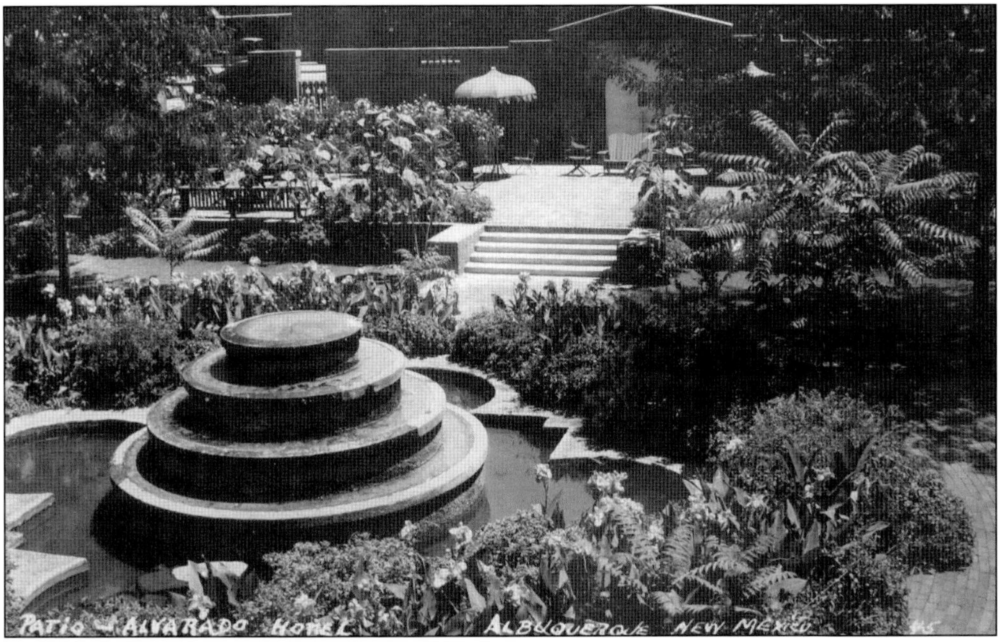

These final views of the Alvarado highlight the garden again and an entrance patio. The lush plantings and quietly dripping fountain must have been especially welcome during the New Mexico summer. The Mission star motif has been carried out in the base form of the fountain, while the wall fountain in the background has a decidedly Roman look. The brick paved courtyard would have been softened when the vines were in leaf. The flattened Mediterranean tile roof is uncharacteristic of both New Mexico and the California missions but certainly sympathetic to the buildings' overall appearance. (Above, courtesy of the UNM CSWR Fred Harvey Collection; below, courtesy of Nancy Tucker.)

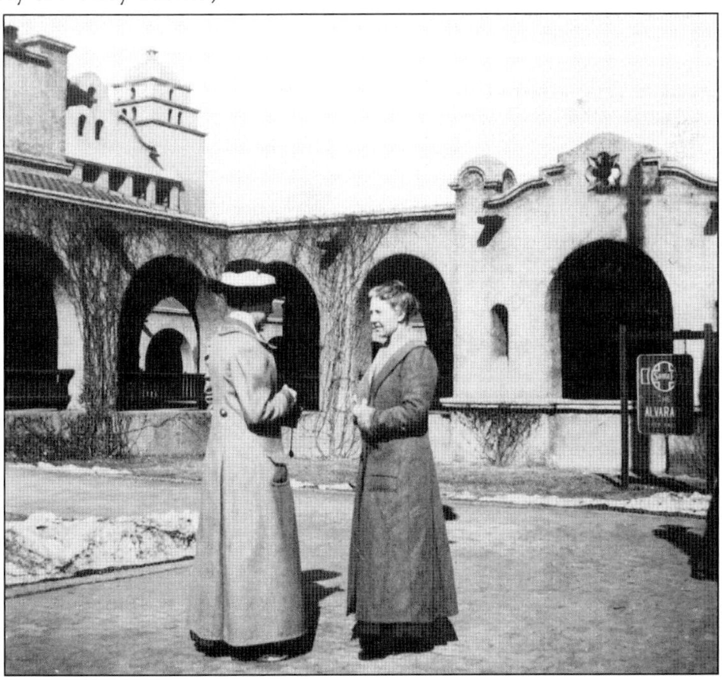

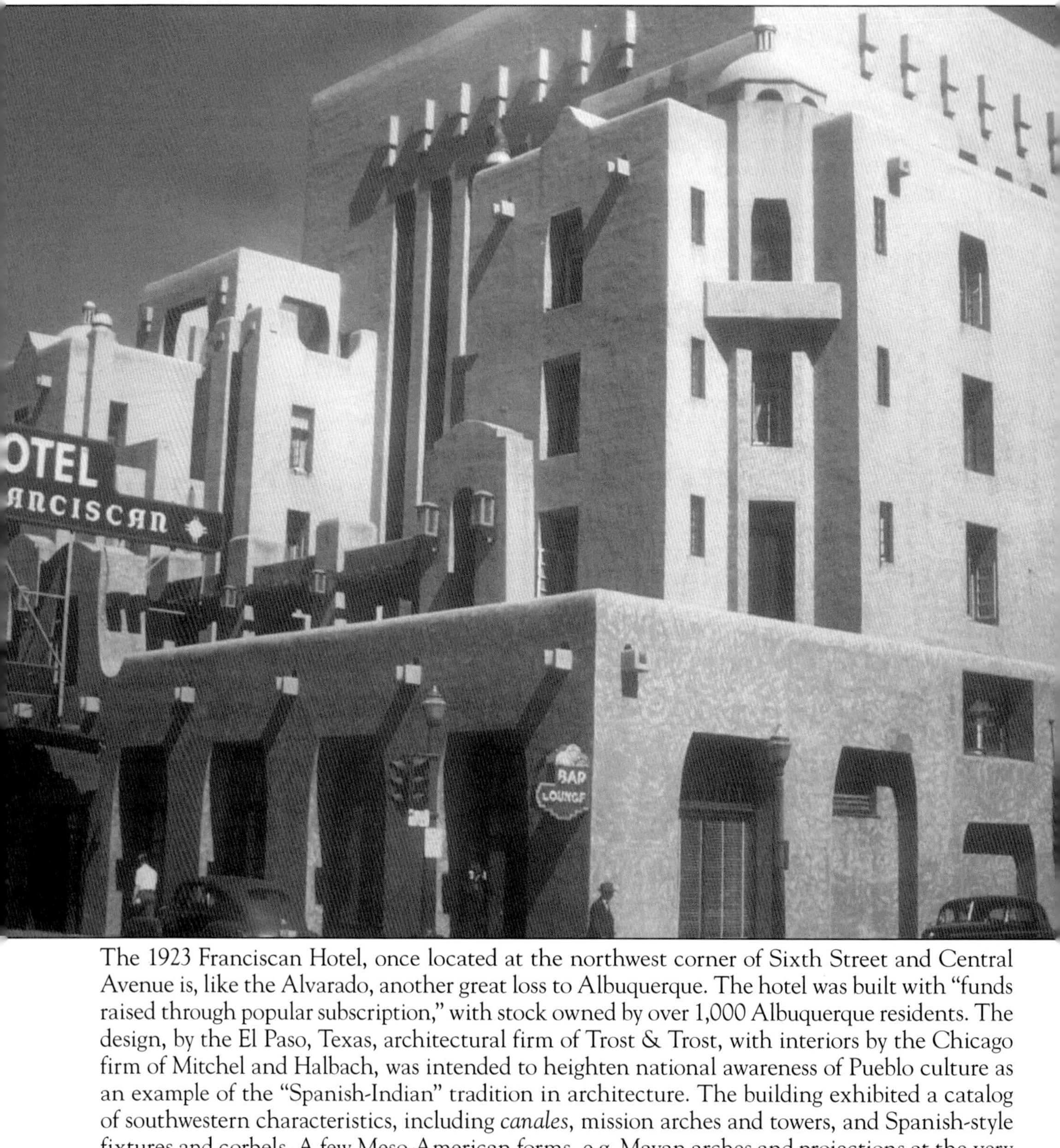

The 1923 Franciscan Hotel, once located at the northwest corner of Sixth Street and Central Avenue is, like the Alvarado, another great loss to Albuquerque. The hotel was built with "funds raised through popular subscription," with stock owned by over 1,000 Albuquerque residents. The design, by the El Paso, Texas, architectural firm of Trost & Trost, with interiors by the Chicago firm of Mitchel and Halbach, was intended to heighten national awareness of Pueblo culture as an example of the "Spanish-Indian" tradition in architecture. The building exhibited a catalog of southwestern characteristics, including *canales*, mission arches and towers, and Spanish-style fixtures and corbels. A few Meso-American forms, e.g. Mayan arches and projections at the very top of the structure, also are apparent. Since the local community was paying for the building, they felt they were justified in influencing the overall design. This was to be a design to celebrate Native American culture and make a tangible statement in opposition to the Department of the Interior Indian Bureau's policy at a time of "liquidating the Indians." (Courtesy of Nancy Tucker.)

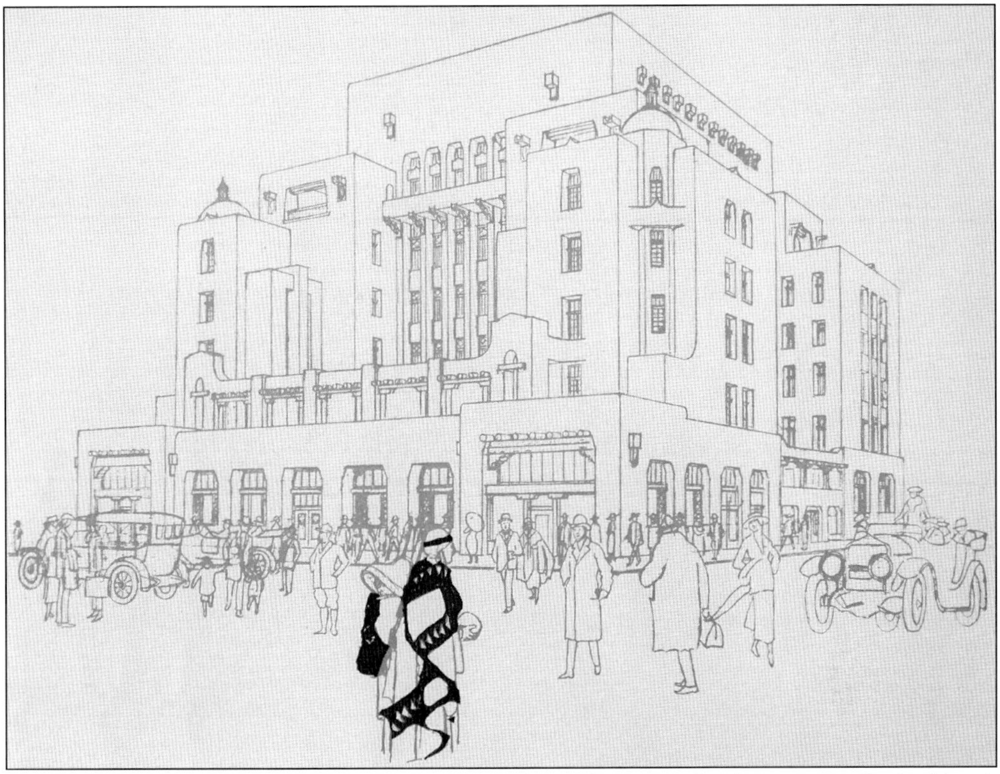

This advertising sketch of the Franciscan from the early 1920s clearly captures the building's dramatic form. The streetscape of Central Avenue, looking east and from the late 1930s, shows the Franciscan as the dominant structure on the west end of the business district with the First National Bank at the other end of the street. The incongruous Greek Temple of the Masons is visible next to the Franciscan on the left side of the photograph. (Both, courtesy of Nancy Tucker.)

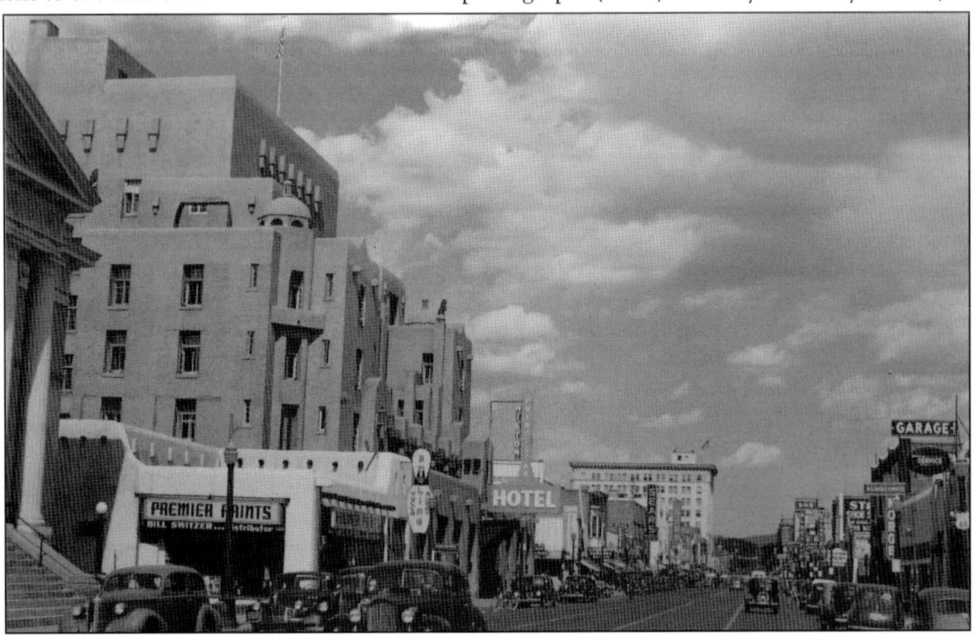

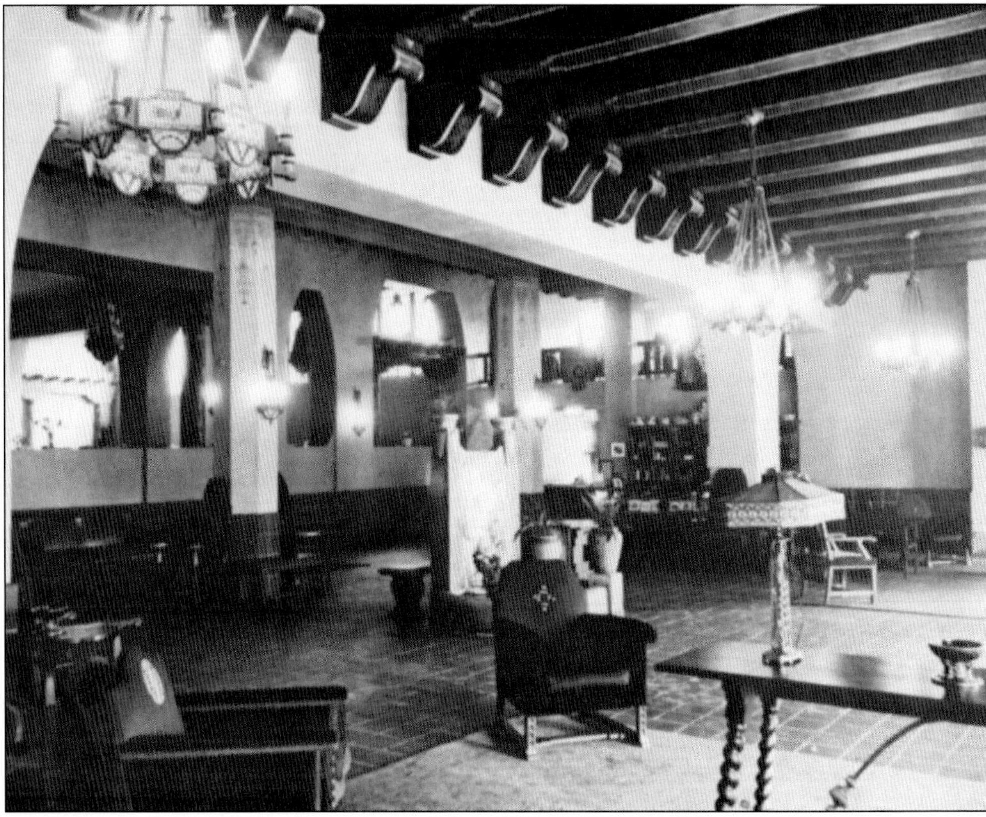

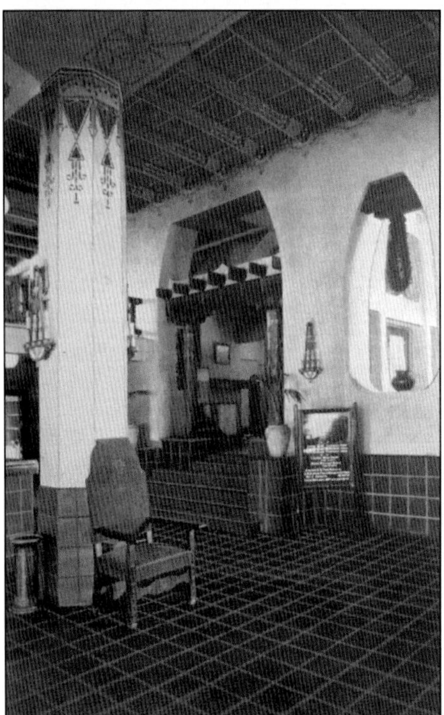

The Franciscan's interiors harmonized with its exterior. Striking Mayan arch forms framed entrances and divided rooms. The strong wall surfaces were broken up by arches and balconies along with carved beams and railings. Navajo rugs were hung from railings, and there were decorative pottery and basket designs stenciled on the walls as border motifs and medallions. These designs were carried over to the heavy ceiling beams. Interior planters and vases softened hard edges. Upholstered chairs, their backs mimicking the shape of arch openings, also added interest to the interior. The interior designs seen here are the work of Inez B. Westlake, who also designed the Franciscan's dishes and stationery. (Both, courtesy of Nancy Tucker.)

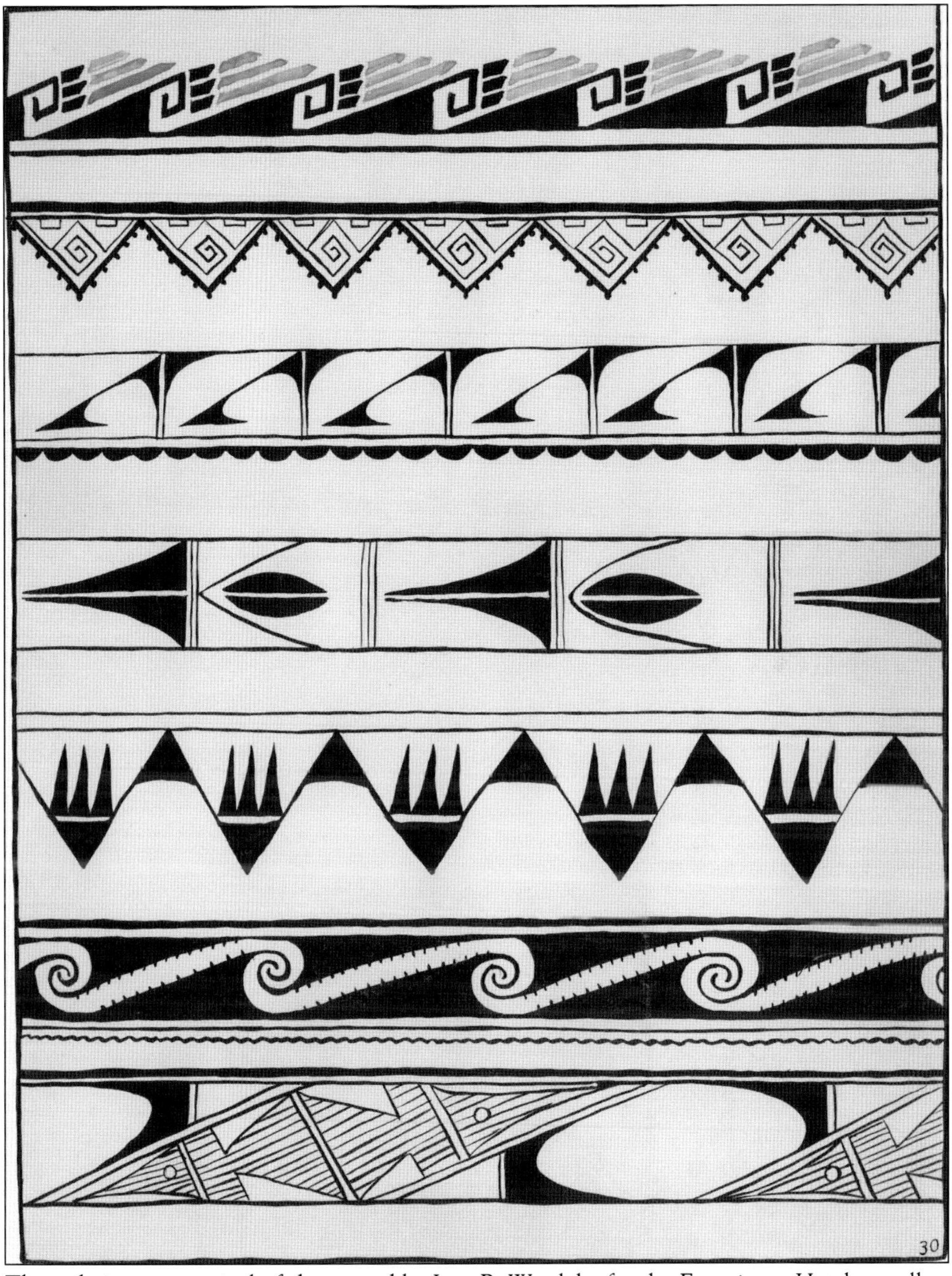

These designs are typical of those used by Inez B. Westlake for the Franciscan Hotel as well as the Kimo Theater (pages 80–87). This is a reproduction of Plate No. 30 from a portfolio entitled *American Indian Designs,* collected and adapted by Inez B. Westlake. The book was published in 1925 by H.C. Perleberg in New York City. The images are, from top to bottom, bead work adapted, modern *hopi*, Indian school Santa Fe, Santo Domingo, *tesuque*, *casas grandes*, and modern Pueblo variations of Old Zuni. (Author's collection.)

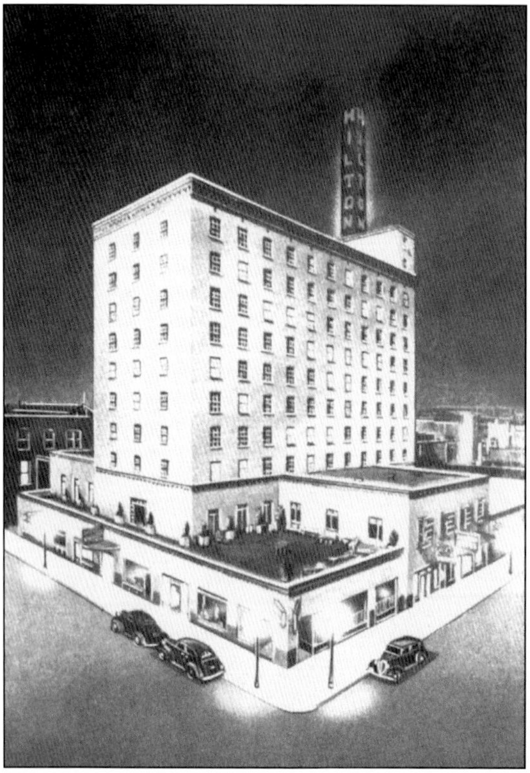

The Hilton Hotel (La Posada, now called the Andaluz), located at the corner of Second Street and Copper Avenue, is 10 stories high with 175 guest rooms. It opened in 1939. It is the sole survivor of the three great Albuquerque hotels. The first two were just reviewed in this chapter. It was Conrad Hilton's fourth hotel and the first modern high-rise hotel in the state. Anton Korn, the hotel's architect, was from Dallas, Texas. He was also known for his single-family residences. A skyscraper box and the two lower floors are Territorial style, i.e. the American New Mexican style of (1846–1880) characterized by a flat roof with brick coping edging the parapet. The original design was Pueblo Revival. (Both, courtesy of Goodman Realty.)

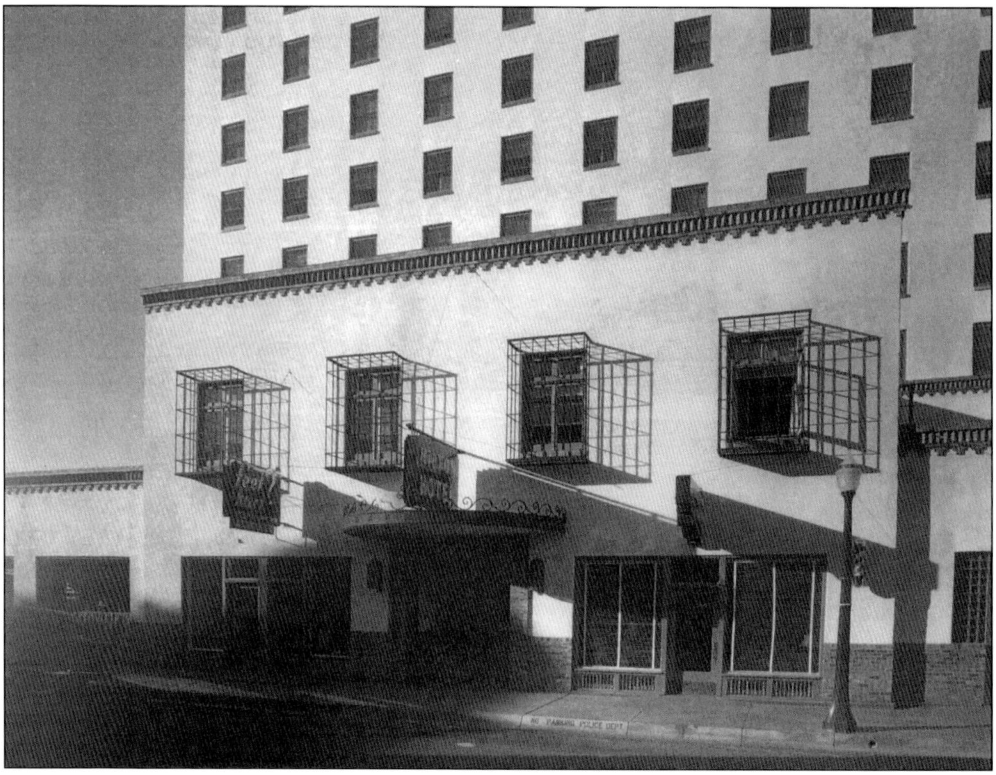

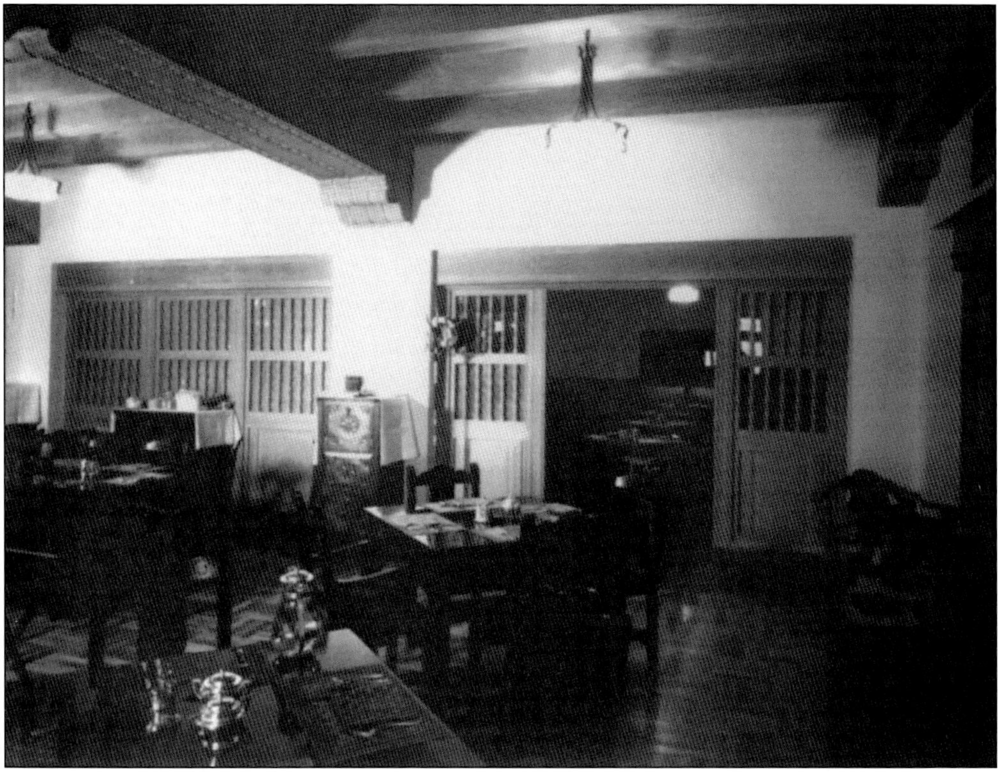

The Hilton's somewhat pedestrian exterior is contrasted by its rich interior. Many of the interior furnishings, artworks, and fixtures were handcrafted by New Mexican artisans. These include carved furniture, tin wall sconces and light fixtures, ironwork and wood carved frames, panels, and ceiling beams. The walls of the dining room as well as several other walls have murals by New Mexican artist Willard Anderson. The hotel opened in time for it to play a role in Albuquerque's growing importance as a military center. A hotel registration card was the only evidence of a meeting between Harry Gold and David Greenglass, which was the basis for the government's case against Julius and Ethel Rosenberg that resulted in their 1953 execution for espionage. (Both, courtesy of Goodman Realty.)

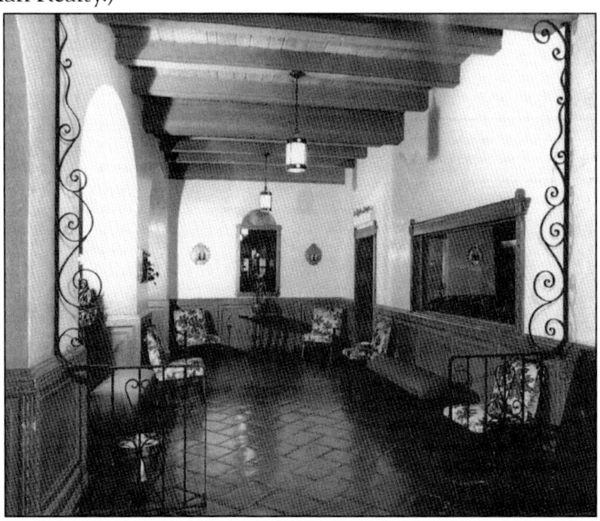

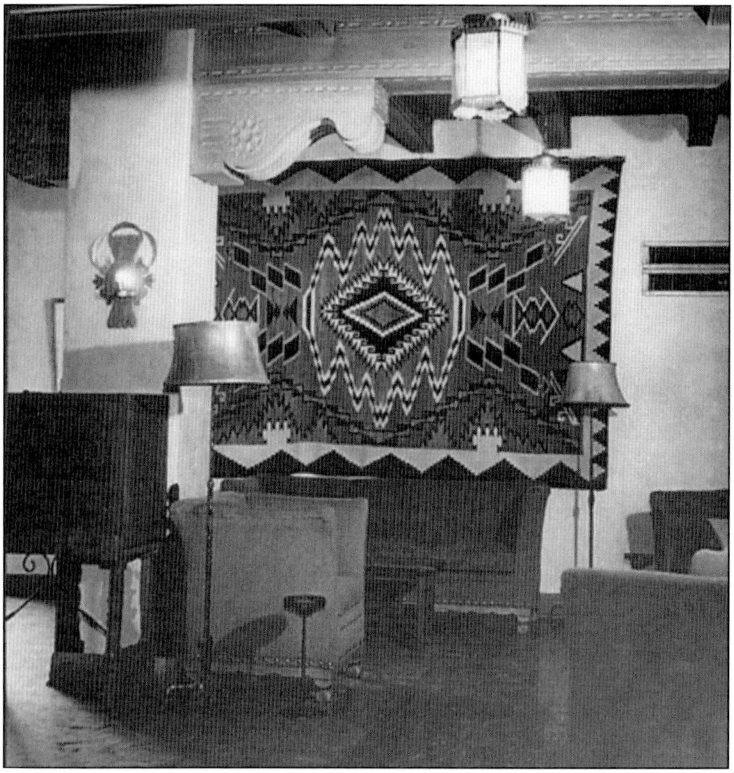

Here are some more interiors of the Hilton, in this case featuring a large and impressive Navajo rug. The carved beams and corbel mirror traditional New Mexican designs, as do the tinwork light fixtures. Hand-carved furniture and handcrafted ironwork is also proximate. (Both, courtesy of Goodman Realty.)

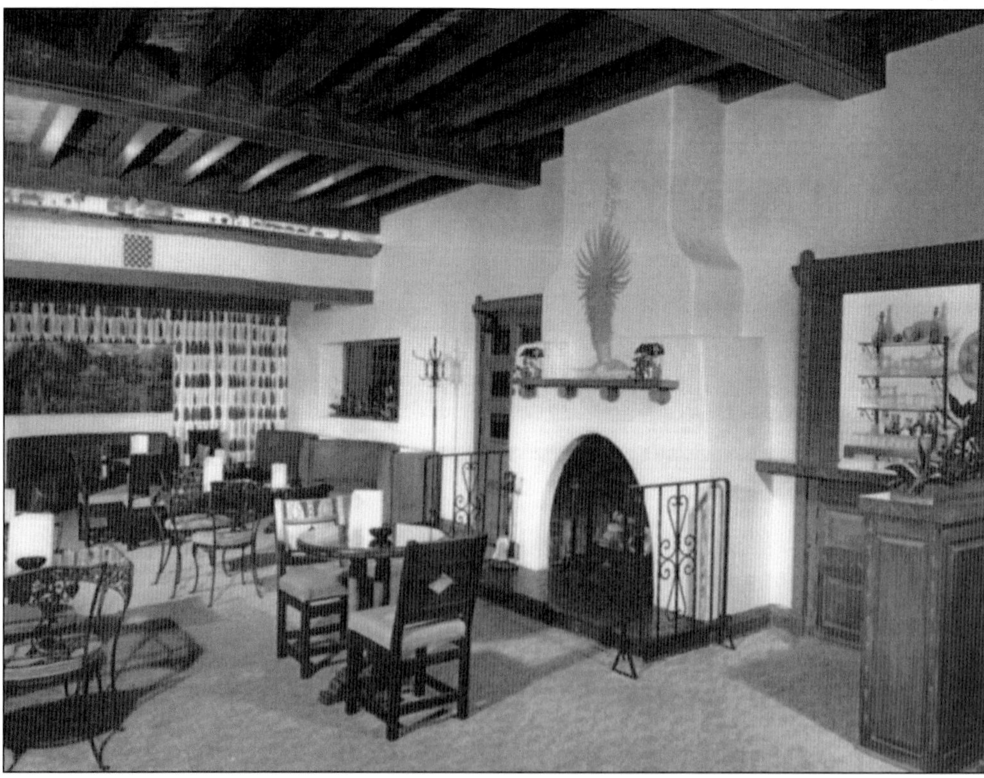

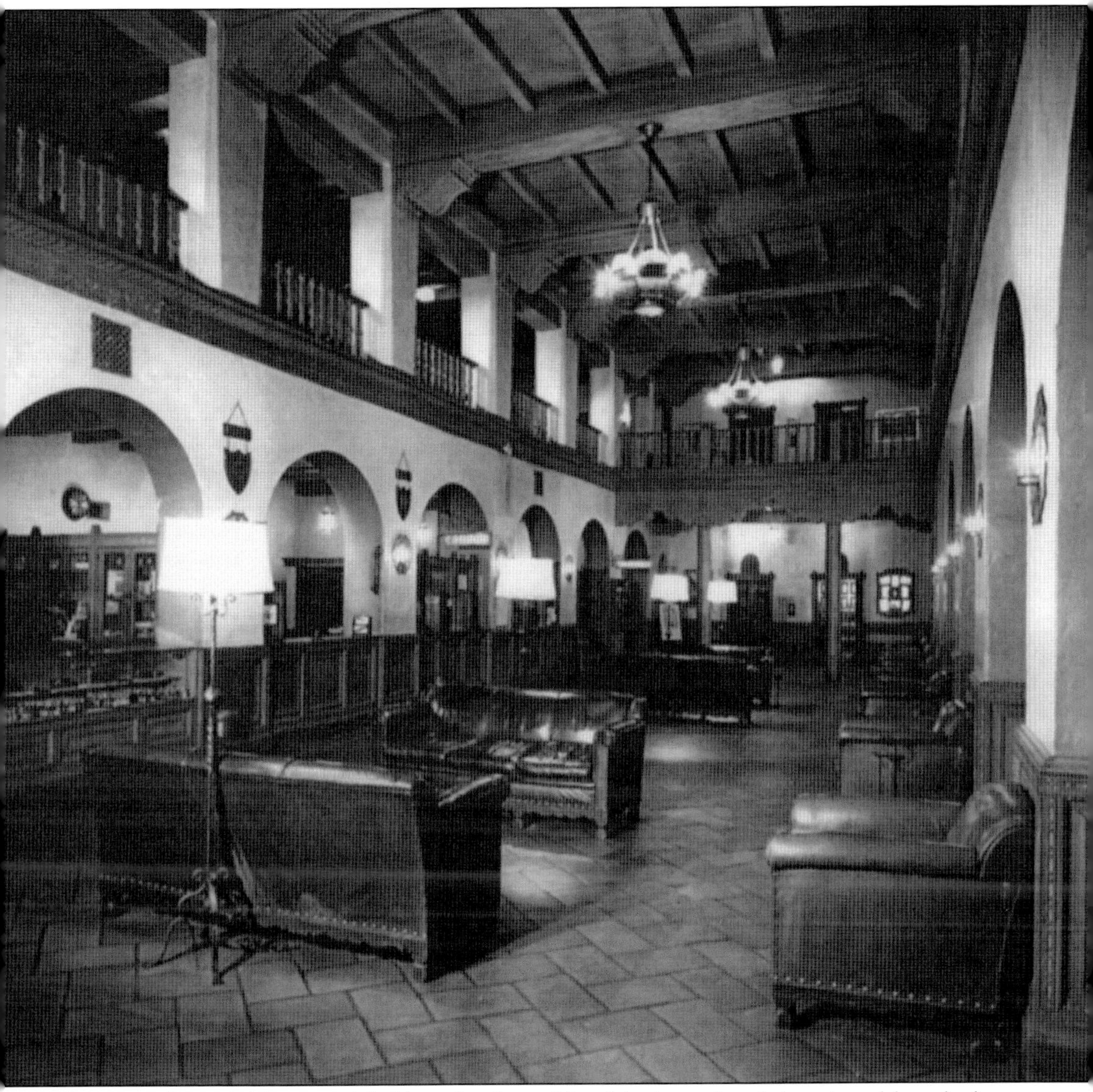

The magnificent lobby is modeled loosely after a New Mexican church interior, although the arched "nave aisles" have more to do with European church architecture then either California or New Mexican churches. The balcony at the end of the lobby looks like a New Mexican choir loft, but here it wraps around one long side, also somewhat like a European church. The simple arches are again reminiscent of the *convento* arches at Isleta (see page 18). And again, it is highly unlikely that there is any direct influence between Isleta and a similar feature found in an entirely different context. (Courtesy of Goodman Realty.)

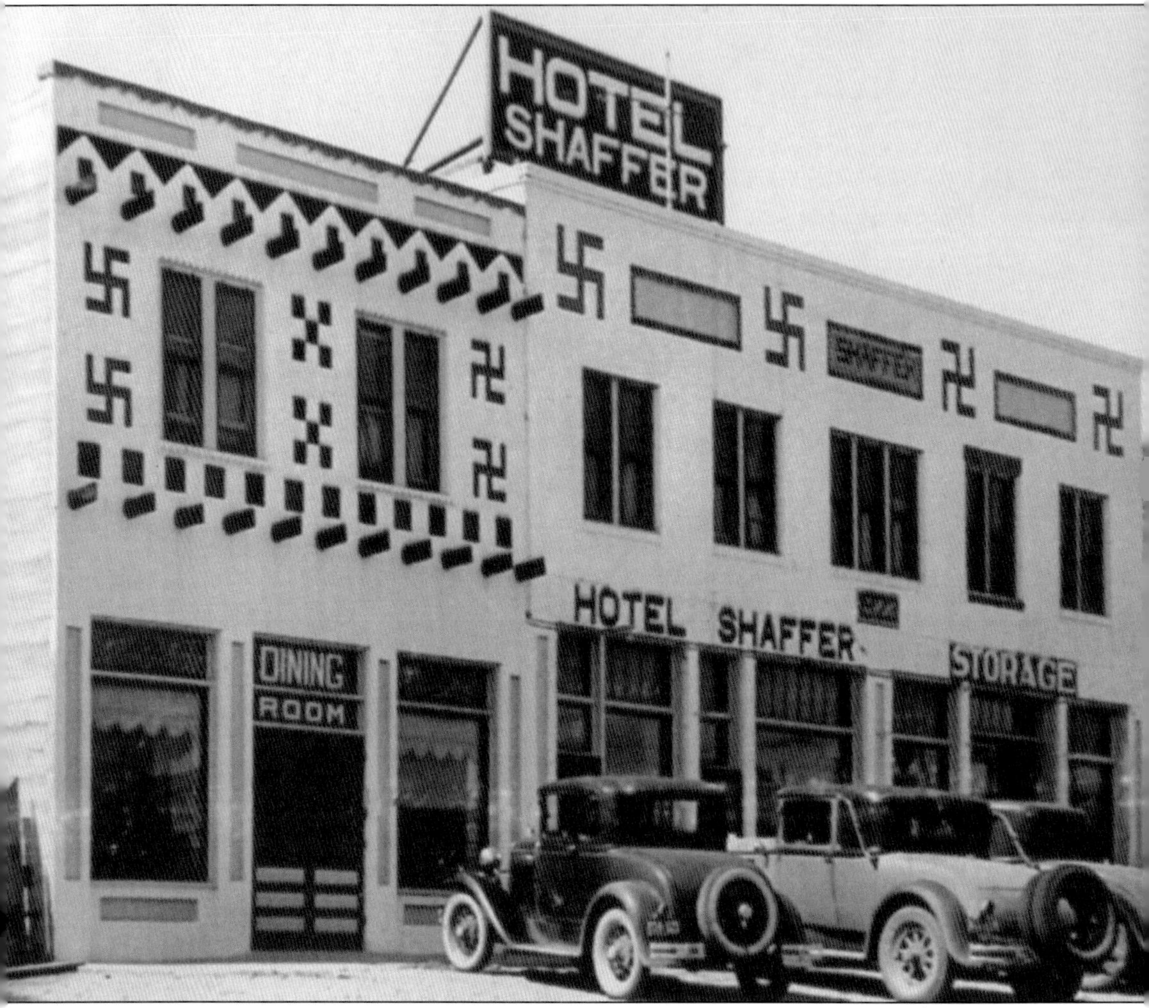

In 1908, Clem "Pop" Shaffer (1880–1964), a blacksmith, came from Indiana to five-year-old Mountainair, the "Pinto Bean Capital of the World." In 1923, a fire destroyed Pop's blacksmith shop and related businesses' structures. He rebuilt in concrete, opened a hotel and dining room on the second floor, and rented the ground floor as a garage. The first-floor walls are one-foot thick, with each wall being a continuous pour. Instead of rebar, the walls are filled with burnt metal from his prior blacksmith and hardware business. The floors are brick. In 1928–1929, he added another building next door, opening a new dining room/restaurant. The Navajo Whirling Logs (i.e., the swastikas, an ancient design found throughout the world; note them also on the light fixtures of the Federal Courthouse, page 30) and other exterior designs, many of which seem to derive from Navajo rugs, were built into the concrete forms. An individualistic work of art and architecture, is it southwestern folk art, Pueblo Deco, Navajo Deco, Coyote Deco, or all four? (Courtesy of the Shaffer Hotel.)

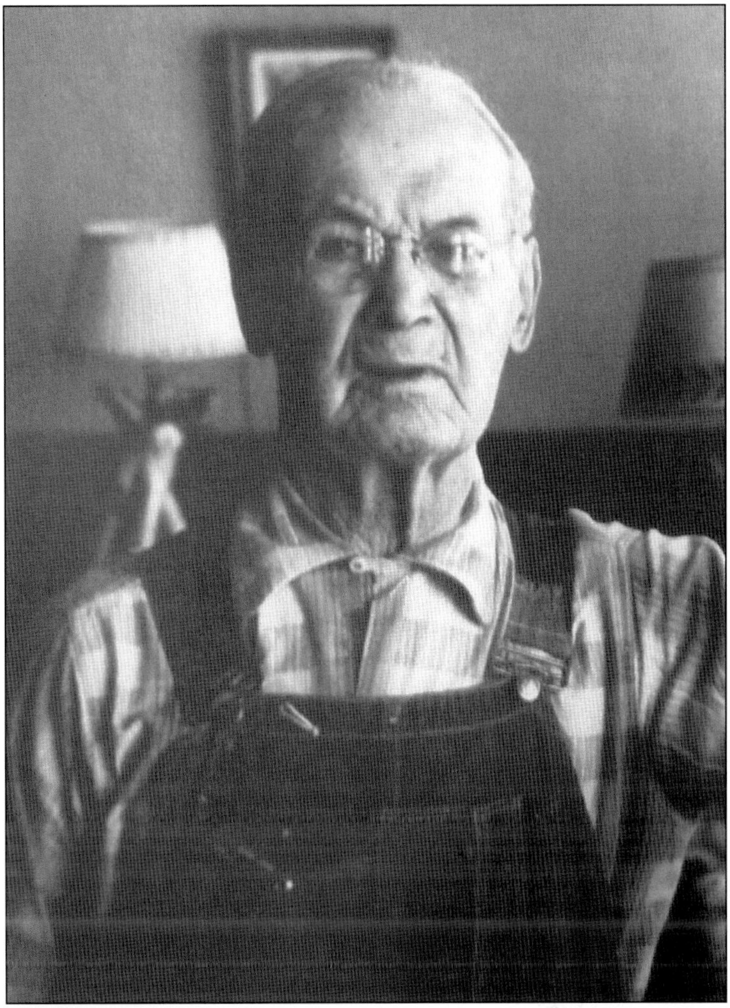

Pop was a "folk artist" who lavished his very personal expression and take on Native American symbolism on his hotel and pretty much everything he touched. In 1937, he established a farm compound called Rancho Bonito that once housed many of his whimsical wooden animal carvings. The carvings ultimately ended up at a tourist stop called The Thing, outside Benson, Arizona. However, a few remain at the Shaffer Hotel. The fence was built in 1931 to enclose the cottage he and his wife, Lena ("Ma"), lived in until it burned. Ernie Pyle said, "You can find in that fence everything in the western hemisphere of the Sears Roebuck Catalogue." (Both, courtesy of the Shaffer Hotel.)

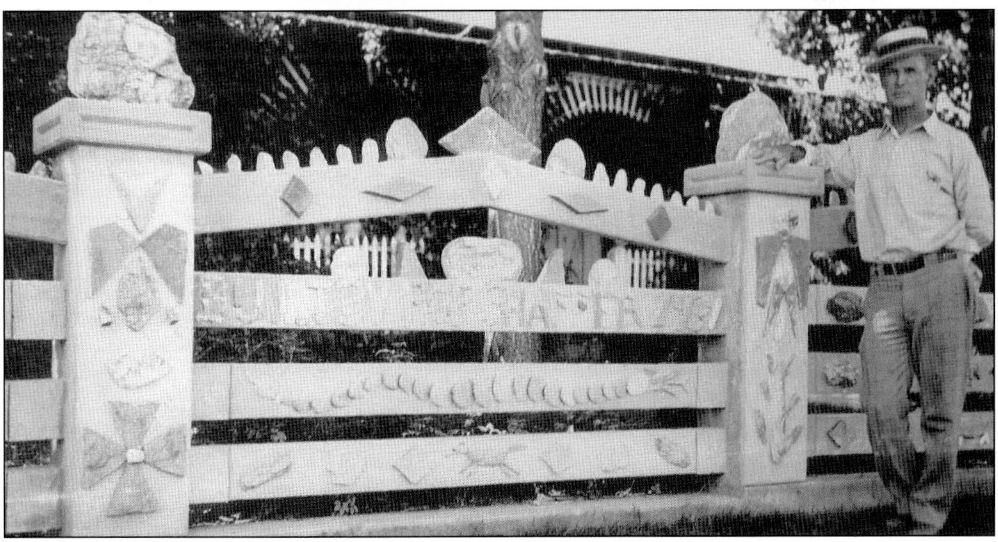

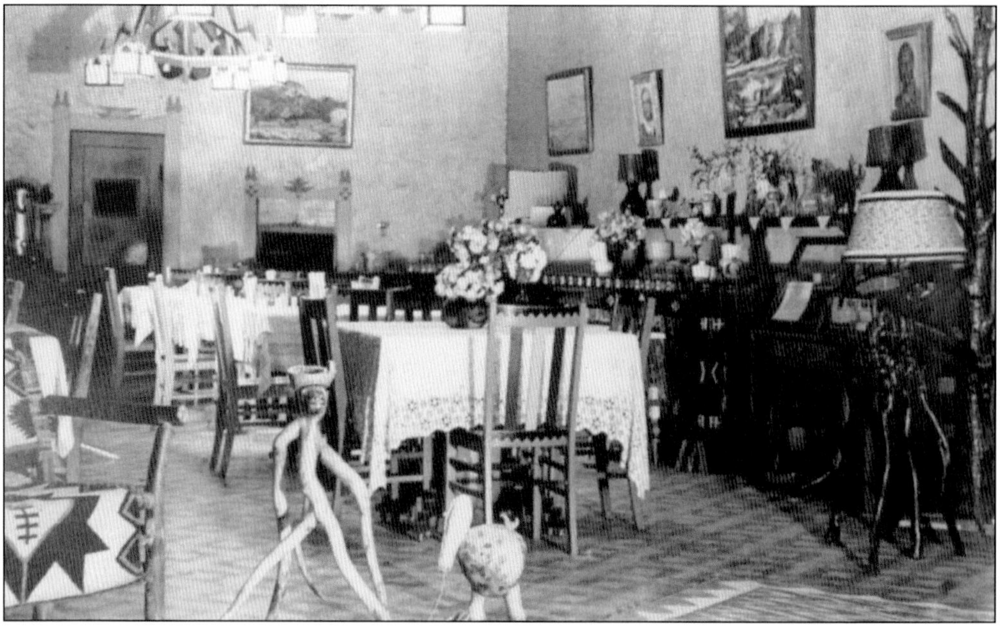

The Shaffer interiors, still intact today, are where Pop's eclectic visions really come to light. The dining room is his masterpiece, and it must be seen in all of its full primary colors to be truly appreciated. Everything in the room bears Pop's hand. He made the light fixtures as well as all the furniture, not to mention the hat rack and the door surrounds. In this picture are even a few of his carved animals. The fireplace bricks are orange, blue, and green with red mortar, probably of Ancho bricks, a nearby brick works that supplied the yellow brick used in the rebuilding of San Francisco following the 1906 earthquake. (Both, courtesy of the Shaffer Hotel.)

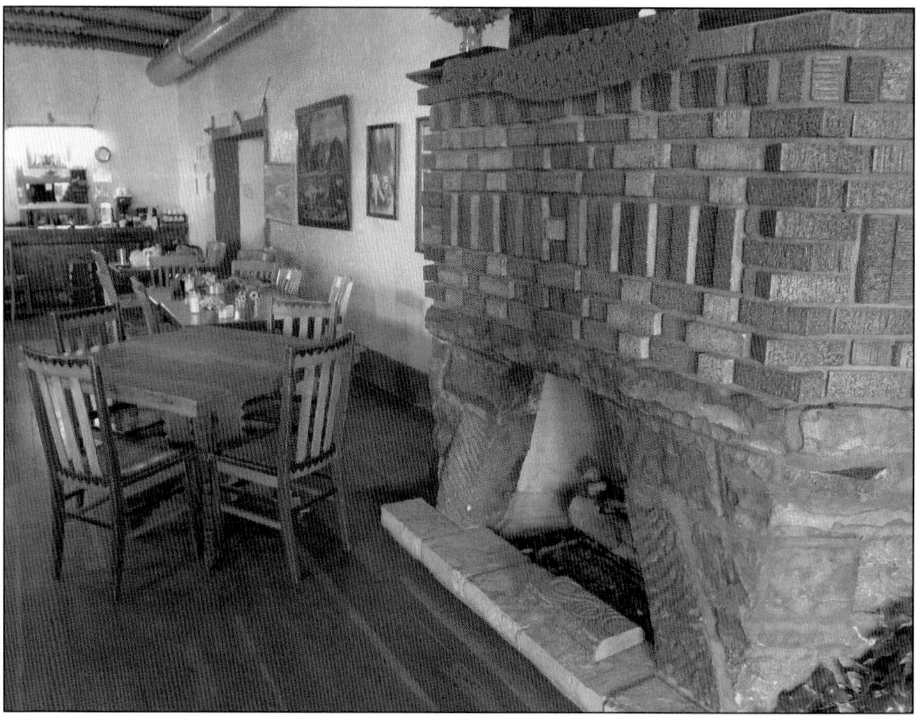

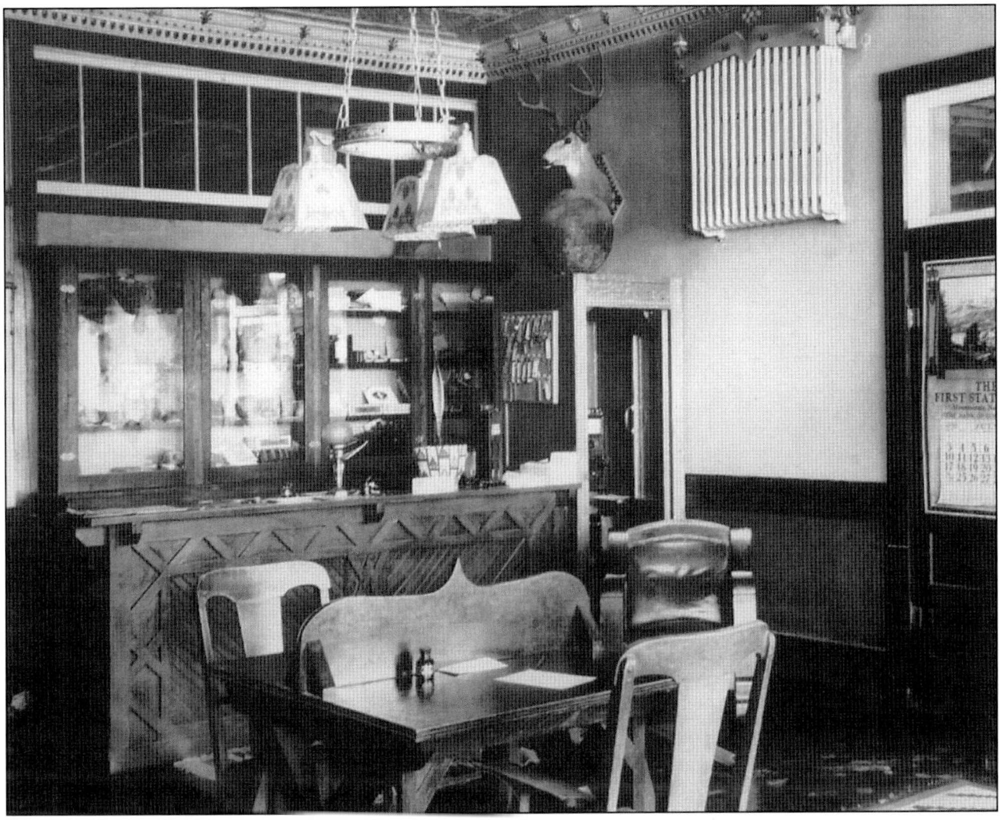

The lobby in the original hotel building is not as elaborate as the dining room, but there is no question as to who built it. Here, the fireplace is composed of dressed native stonework in reds, ochre, and yellow. The design of the front desk repeats themes found throughout the building, as does the cap on the wall-mounted radiator and the hanging light fixture. (Both, courtesy of the Shaffer Hotel.)

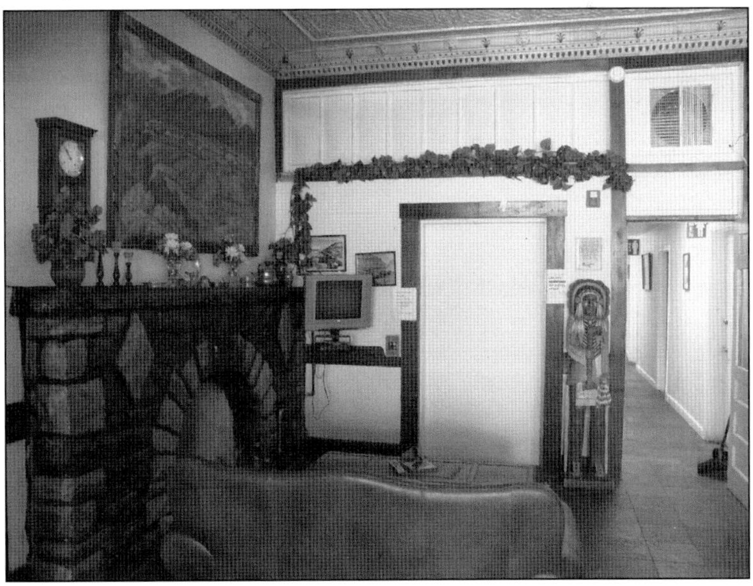

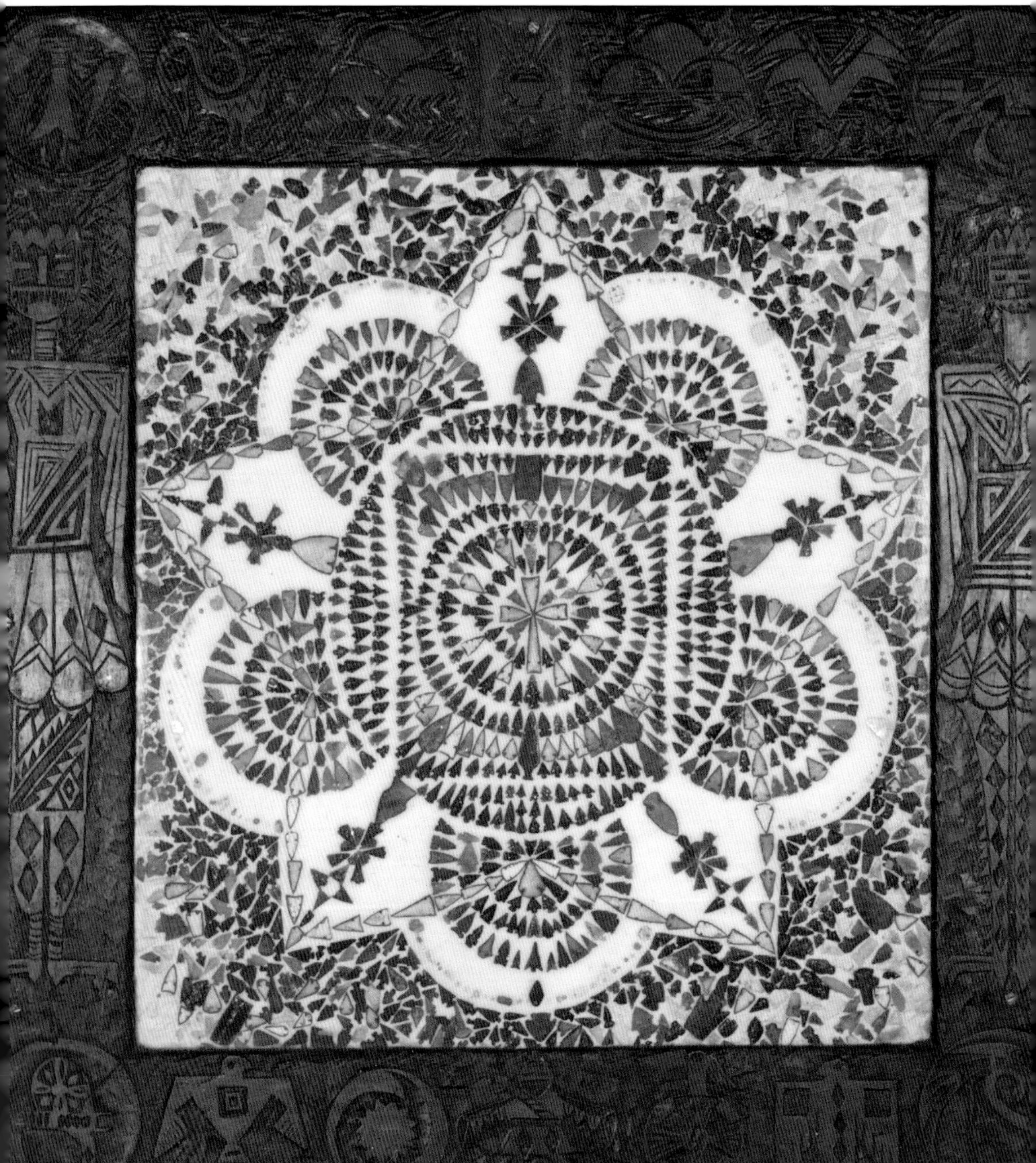

This three-foot square panel is certainly the work of Pop, although where it hung is unknown. It was found as a negative in the Shaffer Hotel archives. The wood carving is a catalog of Pop's ideas of Native American themes. A number of these designs are found on the painted dining room ceiling. They include thunderbirds and pottery designs as well as two fanciful birdmen purely from Pop's imagination. The central design is made entirely from prehistoric projectile points and beads typical of the local area. (Courtesy of the Shaffer Hotel.)

Six

Residences

Pueblo Revival in all of its permutations is, and continues to be, the ubiquitous residential architectural style in Albuquerque and much of New Mexico. A number of books have been written on the subject, so it will only get superficial coverage here. Residential-type buildings were also included in chapter two, specifically University of New Mexico fraternity and sorority houses, and chapter three, especially associated with the VAMC. The Art Deco residential architecture of the city is, however, especially interesting. While it is not widespread, it probably consists of no more than a dozen or so houses, all of which can be categorized as Streamline Moderne, International style, or some combination of the two. If they have curves, then they can be called Streamline, and if they are entirely rectilinear, then they are International. The massing of these houses has been clearly influenced by the Pueblo Revival, most being a series of low cubes reminiscent of Pueblo forms, perhaps with a curved room or window. Four such structures that provide a clear idea of the type are included in this chapter. All of these houses still exist, although some have been extensively modified or are hidden by walls and landscaping. The exception is the magnificent Lembke House, which though tastefully expanded, remains completely exposed on its corner lot. Finding contemporary photographs of these older houses proved a challenge. Several came from snapshots originally used in *Albuquerque Progress* magazine, a booster publication of the Albuquerque National Trust and Savings Bank and the best source of building information from the mid-1930s through the 1950s.

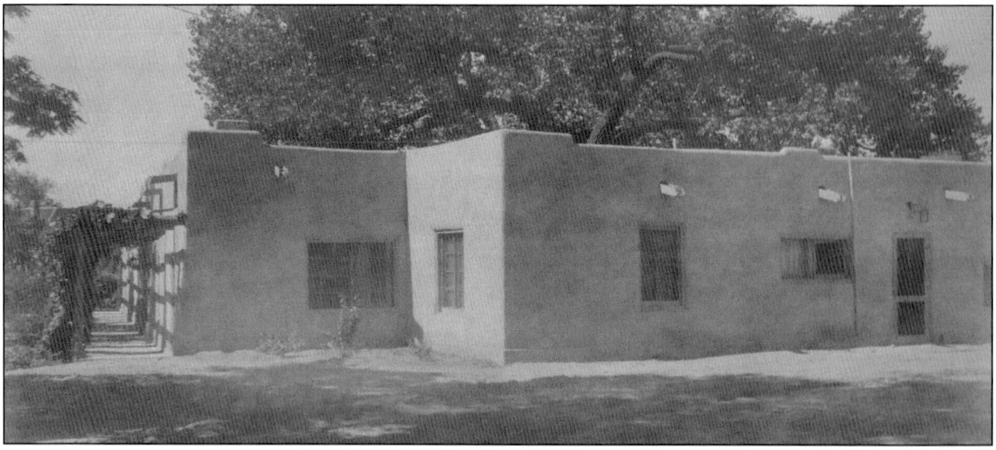

Erna Fergusson (1888–1964) was an avid writer, historian, and storyteller who documented the culture and history of New Mexico for more than 40 years. Her 1922 house represents the Pueblo type in its classic form and is a reflection of the "old" Albuquerque she celebrated in her writings. (Courtesy of UNM CSWR, Special Collection Department, Erna Fergusson House.)

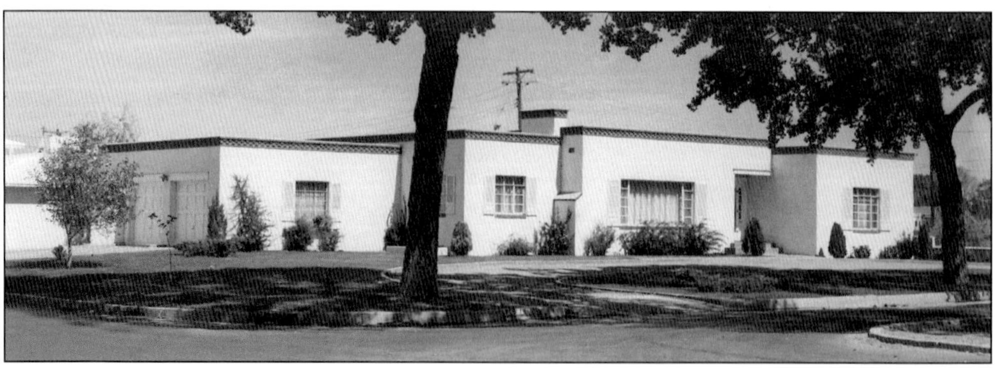

Although the brick parapet is pure Territorial style, the windows say, "International style," with no hint of Greek Revival pediments. This well-proportioned house, of unknown date and architect, is located at the northwest corner of San Cristobal Road and Laguna Boulevard. (Courtesy of the Albuquerque Museum.)

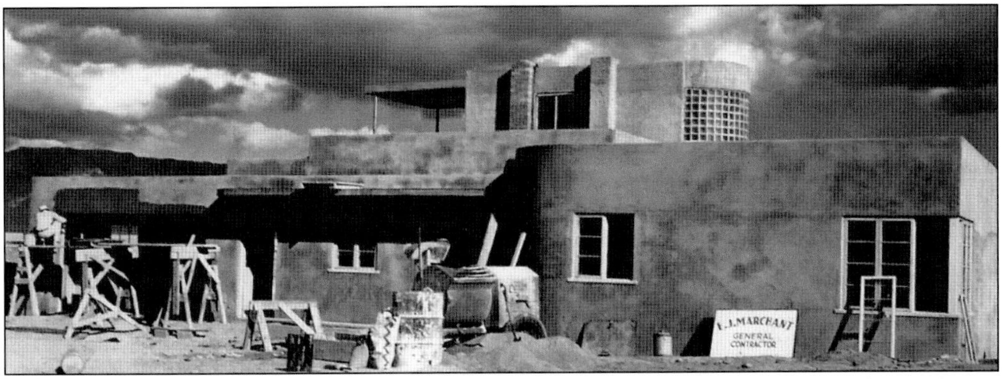

The two-bedroom Kelvin (or Kelvinator) house completed in 1938 was a speculative design promoted by the Raabe and Mauger Hardware Company. The Streamline Moderne house was designed as a "Machine for Living" and described as an "ultra-modern, electrically equipped, air-conditioned home." The design of William Burk Jr. was meant to demonstrate that modern did not need to be expensive. It has been well maintained in near original condition. (Courtesy of the Albuquerque Planning Department.)

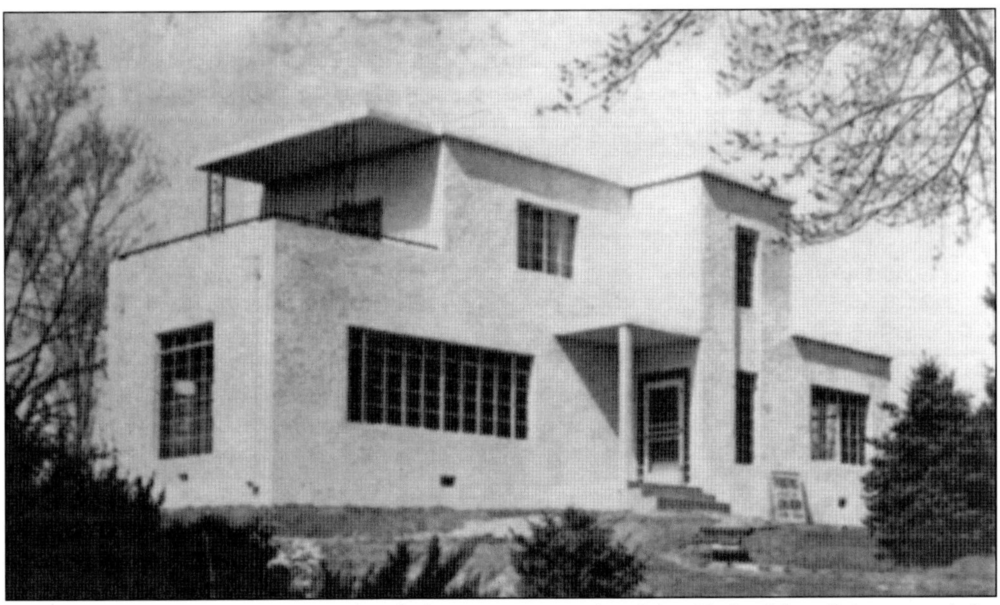

In March 1940, this International-style house was completed for Clyde Odin. Odin owned the city's Buick dealership, served on the state highway commission, and became Albuquerque's mayor in 1930. His large house would have been seen as one of the most modern in the city. (Courtesy of *Albuquerque Progress* magazine.)

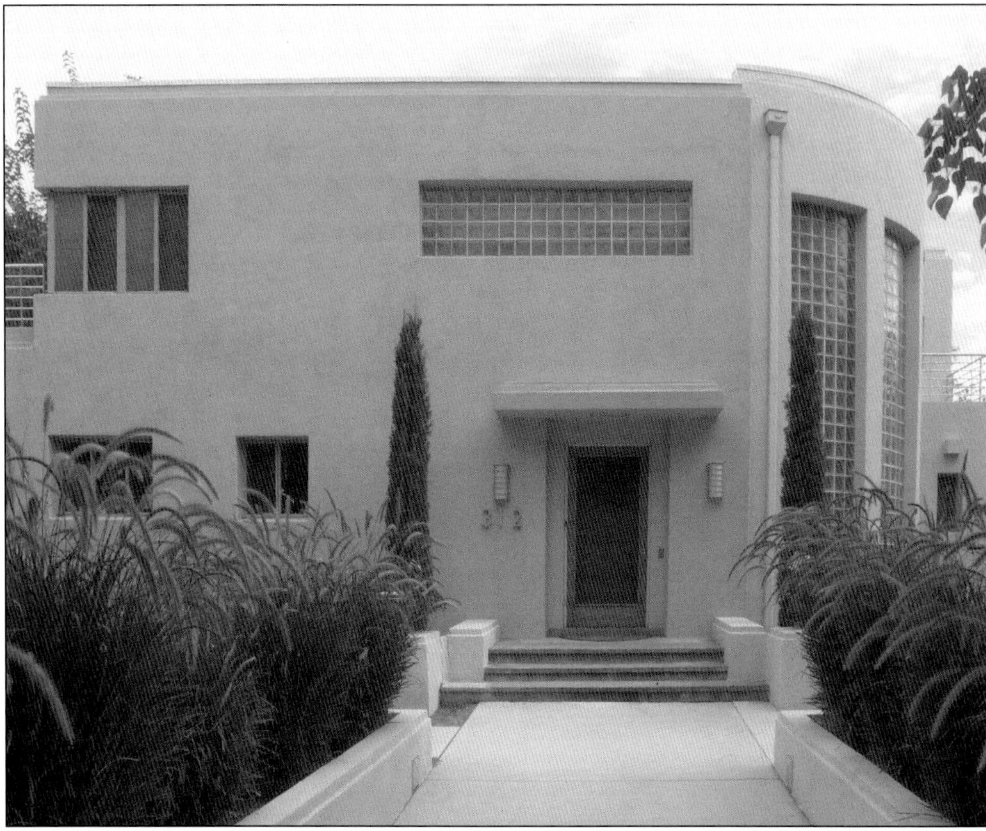

The 1937 Lembke House embodies characteristics of both the International style and Streamline Moderne (see chapter one on page 16). It was one of the few houses in the Huning Castle neighborhood built during the Depression. The house was designed by Townes and Funk of Amarillo, Texas, and was constructed as a speculative venture by building contractor Charles Lembke (see a similar building on page 67). (Author's collection.)

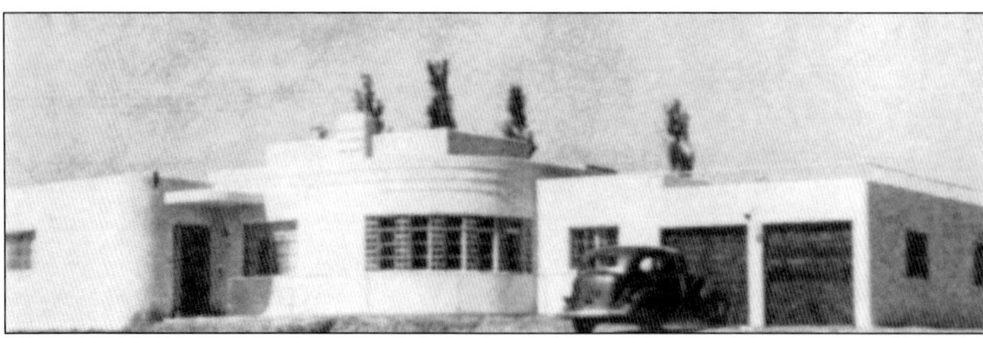

Completed in mid-1938, this fine Streamline Moderne house was built for Walter J. Kavanaugh, the manager of Given Bros. Shoes (see page 69). Compare this single-story composition to the nearby Kelvin house on the previous page. The blocky form is reminiscent of the Pueblo style, but with no *vigas*, glass bricks, and round corners, it becomes Moderne. (Courtesy of the Albuquerque Planning Department, *Albuquerque Progress* magazine.)

Seven

The Maisel Murals

The lengthy murals fronting Maisel's are one of the few examples of Native American workmanship on a building. They are the prominent statement of the structure's front facade and harmonize well with the simplified Art Deco detailing of metalwork and black glass panels of the entry. Architect Meem contracted with important Santa Fe artist Olive Rush, who painted three of the murals. Rush altered her initial assignment by subcontracting work to Dorothy Dunn of the Santa Fe Indian School (SFIS). Dunn had established The Studio of art instruction at SFIS in 1932 and ran the program until 1937. She influenced a generation of Native American painters. J.J. Brody in *Indian Painters and White Patrons* wrote, "The Studio of the SFIS became the first programmed art training center for Indians. It attempted to encourage individual patterns of growth through the use of modern techniques." SFIS also demanded a strict tribal orientation of its students. Through art, Dunn intended to engender respect for cultural traditions and instill individual pride and accomplishment. Kenneth Chapman of the School of American Research and a founder of the Indian Arts Fund became her advisor. For the Maisel murals, she hired several of the former SFIS students at $150 each for two weeks of work in early 1939. The Maisel murals are a "who's who" of Navajo and Pueblo artists since essentially all of them became famous in their own right. High-quality *cassien tempura*, a gluey medium made from curdled milk, was used to paint the murals and was provided by Dunn. The murals, although cracked and somewhat soiled, remain in original unrestored condition, with generally bright colors and no loss of the painted surface. "We were real young and inexperienced . . . I was so broke. I needed the money," said Pabilita Velarde of Santa Clara Pueblo, one of the muralists. "We joked around a lot during the job. Mr. Maisel came out quite often, gave us encouraging words. He gave us coffee and milk and soda pop," said Joe Herrera, another one of the muralists. Artist Pop Chalee become so engrossed with the work of others that, not paying attention, she fell off the scaffolding but was fortunately not seriously injured.

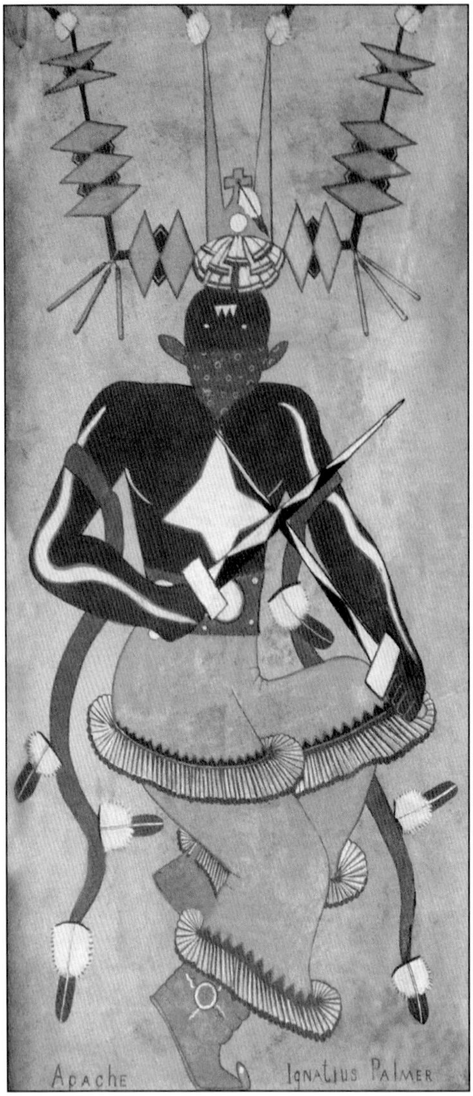

This mural is called *Apache Gan Dancer* by Ignatius Palmer, a Mescalero Apache (1922–present). The *gan* ("mountain spirits") once lived with humans but are now immortal supernatural beings associated with certain mountains and caves. They are an important presence in girls' puberty rites. Palmer is a very competent painter, with work in several major museum collections, and worked for many years as a repairman for the Bureau of Indian Affairs in Albuquerque. (Courtesy of Skip Maisel.)

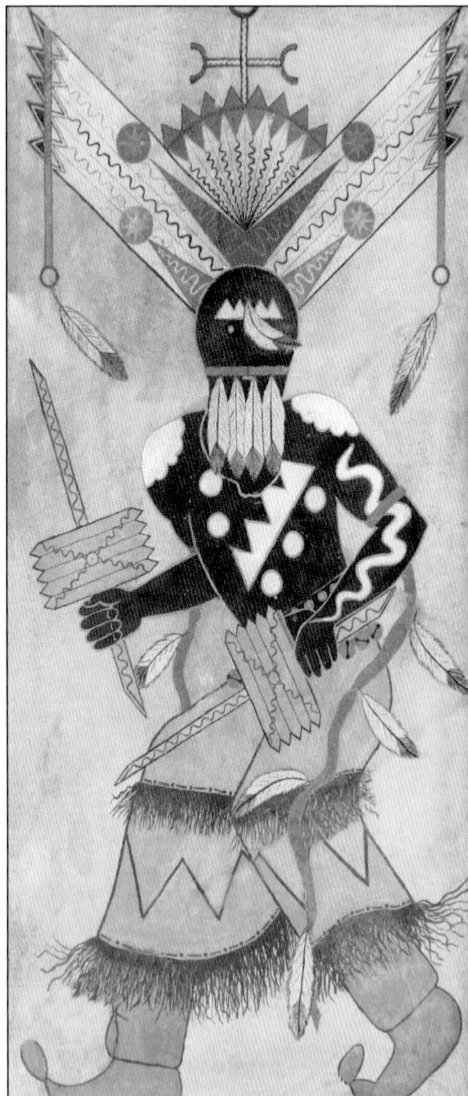

This mural is titled *Apache Gan Dancer* by Wilson Dewey, also called Sundust, a San Carlos Apache (1915–1969). "Palmer succeeded in evoking the characteristic stomp, twist and stop-short action of the dance pattern [while] Dewey's figures were done in a quieter mood," wrote Dorothy Dunn. Dewey was a student at the Santa Fe Indian School for three years beginning in 1935. He finished his final year of education at the Albuquerque Indian School. (Courtesy of Skip Maisel.)

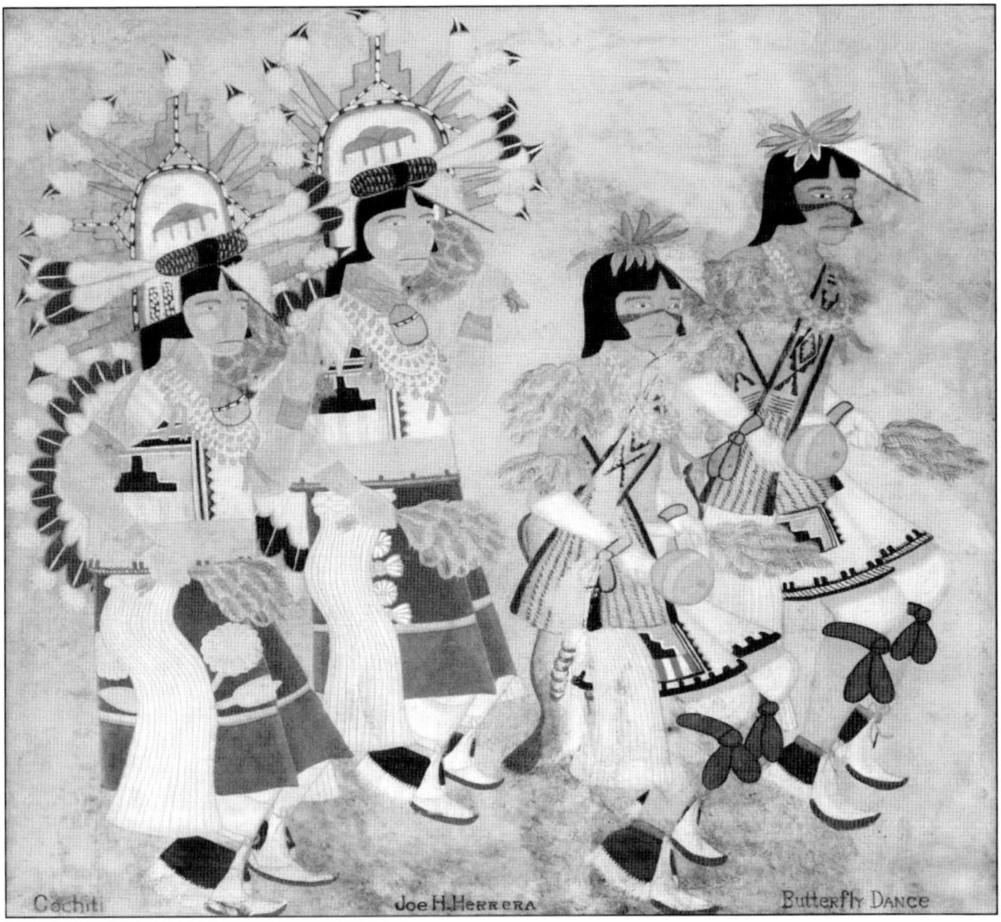

The above mural is called *Butterfly Dance with Four Dancers* by See Ru/Joe H. Herrera, from Cochiti Pueblo (1923–2001). On the right is *Butterfly Maiden* by Popovi Da/Tony Martinez, from San Ildefonso Pueblo (1923–1971). Popovi Da is the son of famous potter Maria Martinez (see following page). Herrera is the son of a famous painter, Tonita Pena. He learned his mother's technique, but his style is more sensitive and with a finer feeling for color and line than his mother. The Butterfly Dance is a social dance and a popular theme with Herrera. It may relate to a Cochiti tale concerning the pursuit of a butterfly by two young girls who try to catch the butterfly to use the wing pattern for pottery designs. Note the corn and rain symbols on the headdresses (*tablita*) of the two women in the Herrera painting. (Both, courtesy of Skip Maisel.)

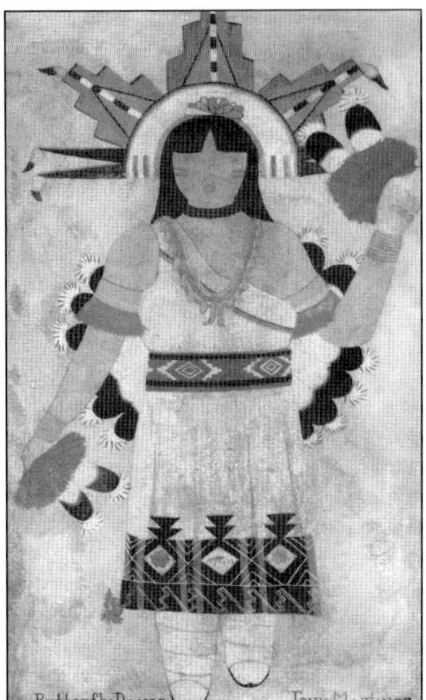

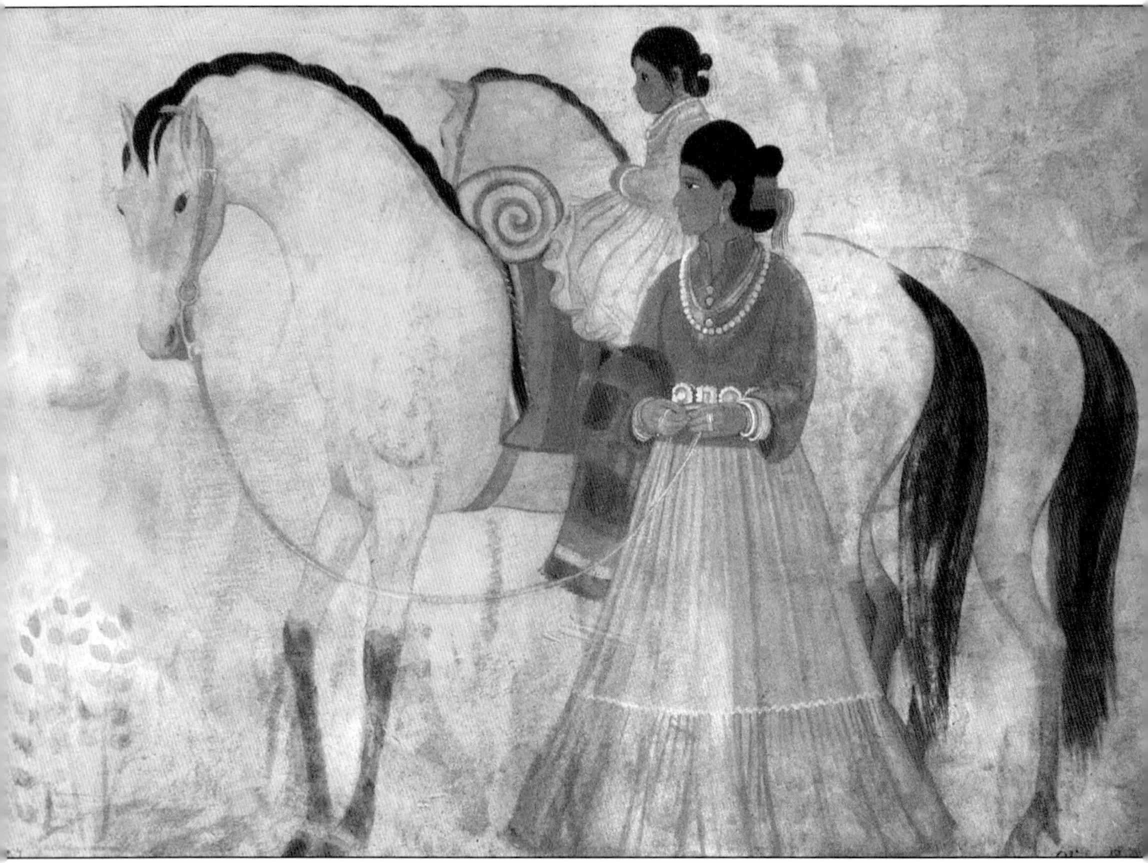

This mural, called *Navajo Women on Horseback* by Olive Rush (1873–1966), depicts a scene from Navajo daily life. Olive Rush was born in Fairmont, Indiana, and following several visits to New Mexico, settled permanently in Santa Fe in 1920. She was a well-known illustrator and muralist and an important influence in Native American art education. The Maisel murals were her last Native American art project, a project where she worked alongside the other artists. (Courtesy of Skip Maisel.)

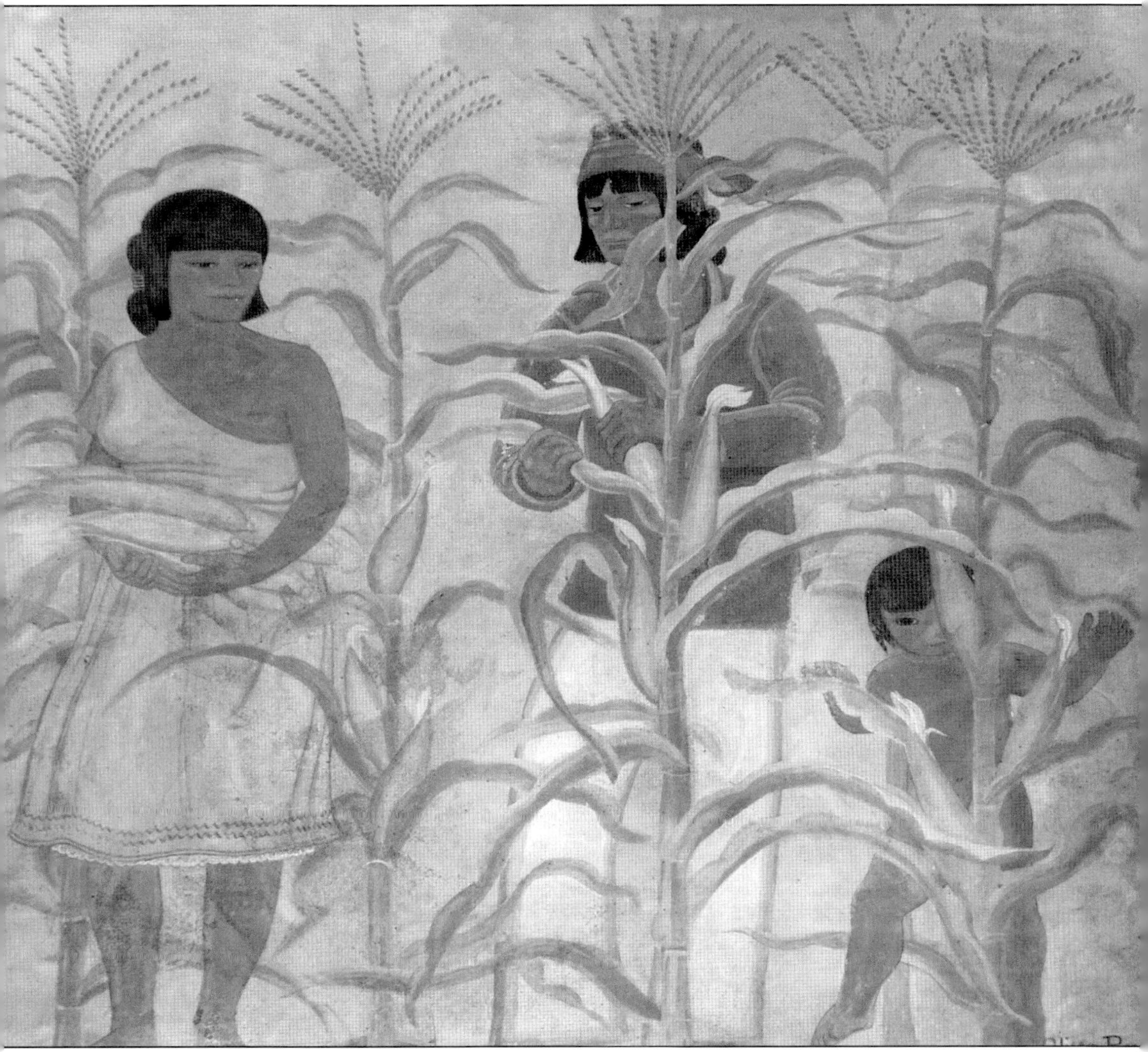

This mural is called *Gathering Corn* by Olive Rush (1873–1966) and pictures a scene from Pueblo daily life. Rush selected the individuals to paint the murals, several of whom were students at the Santa Fe Indian School, as well as providing paint and guidance. Pablita Velarde described her as follows: "She was very feminine—soft-spoken and almost fragile. All of her work had that soft tone with hidden messages. Hers was a great spirit." (Courtesy of Skip Maisel.)

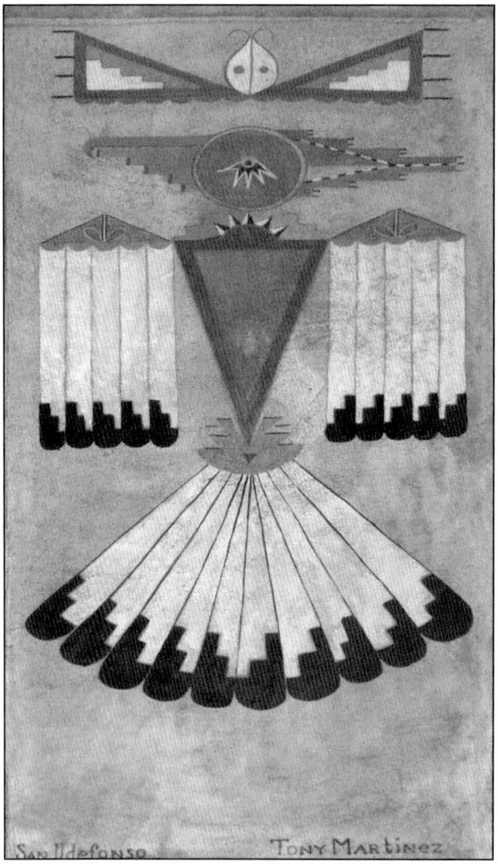

This mural is called *Rain Birds* by Popovi Da/ Tony Martinez, from San Ildefonso Pueblo (1923–1971). His family includes a number of famous artists, the most prominent being his parents, potters Julian and Maria Martinez. He served as the governor of San Ildefonso Pueblo and ran a gallery to promote his mother's pottery. Dorothy Dunn described him as an inventive, clean, and classic painter. The rain bird is a common Pueblo symbol, often seen as a painted pottery design. H.P. Mera, in his discussion of the Rain Bird motif, states that "In tracing the ancestry of the Rain Bird design it will be necessary to go back to the very beginnings of decorated pottery in the Southwest." The two birds depicted here are very similar in style, yet strikingly different in feeling. (Courtesy of Skip Maisel.)

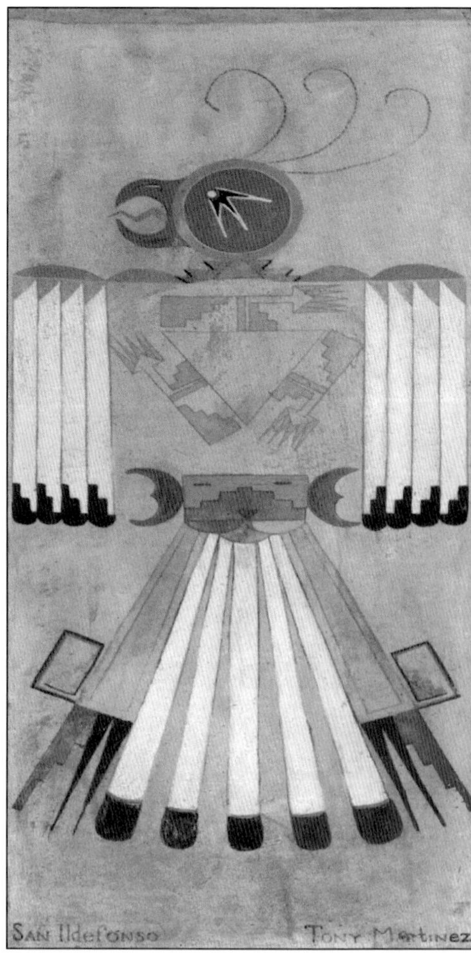

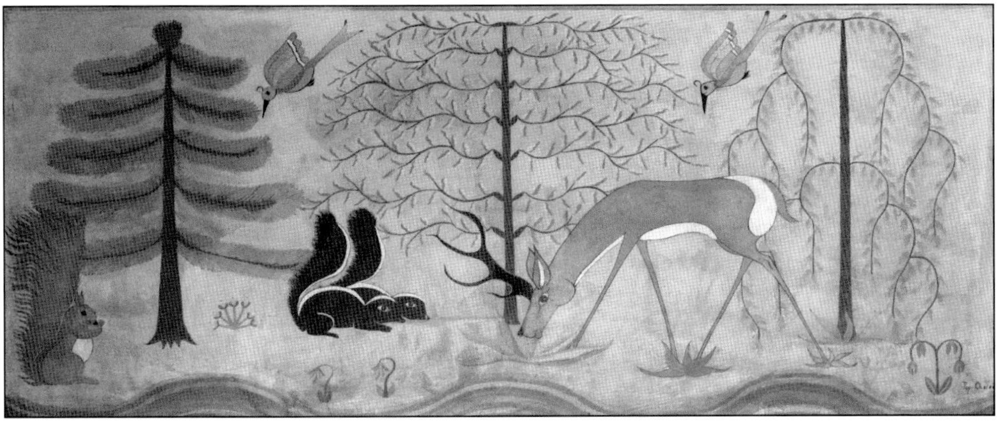

This mural is called *Animals in the Forest* by Pop Chalee/Merina Lujan Hopkins (1908–1993). Chalee was born in Castle Gate, Utah, to a Taos father and an East Indian mother. She was an accomplished muralist who produced art for TWA air terminals and Marshall Field's department store in Chicago. She, along with Harrison Begay, worked for Walt Disney on the 1942 production of *Bambi*. Her whimsical forest animals in a mythic landscape shown here clearly relate to the later Disney work. The *Deer Dancers* depicted by Olive Rush (1873–1966) are part of the Rio Grande Pueblo winter ceremonials associated with hunting. They often appear in a group along with elk, buffalo, antelope, and mountain sheep impersonators. It is interesting to contrast Rush's rather Oriental deer with Chalee's cartoon deer, as both artists were influenced by Oriental art. (Courtesy of Skip Maisel.)

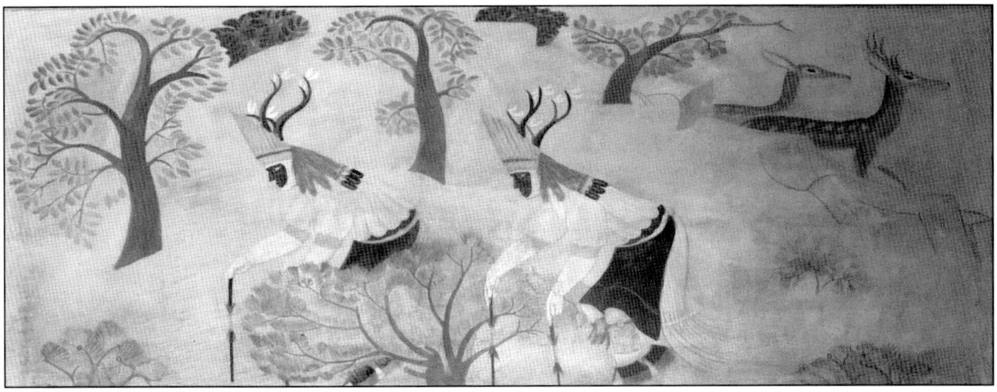

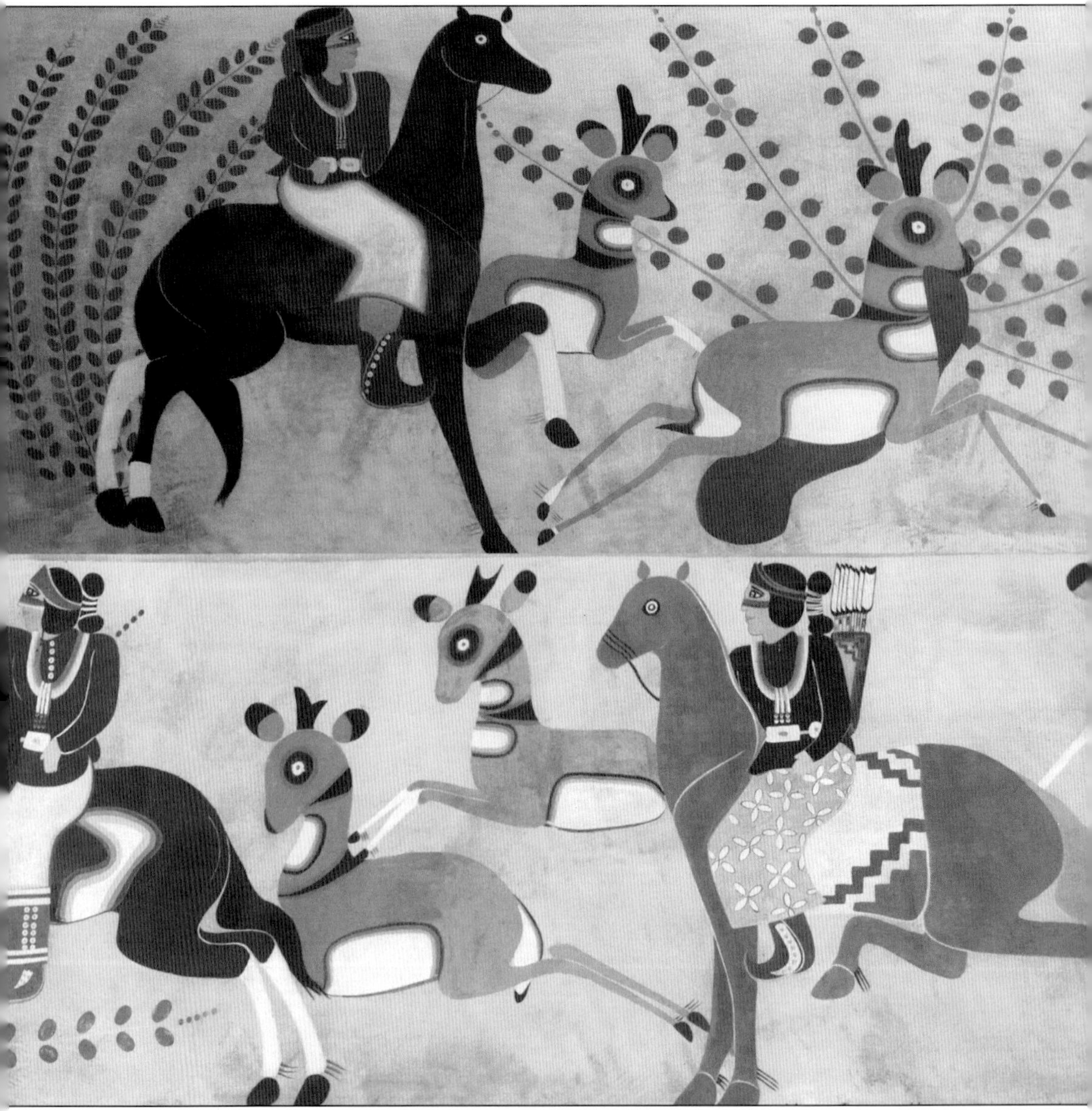

This mural is called *Navajo Ceremonial Hunt* by Ha-so-de/Narciso "Ciso" Platero Abeyta, a Navajo from Cañoncito, now Tóhajiilee, New Mexico (1918–1998). The largest of the Maisel murals, this depiction of a ceremonial antelope hunt is by perhaps the most individualistic and expressive of any of the artists to come out of the Santa Fe Indian School Studio. Three male riders on the left and center, along with two female riders on the right, chase down a herd of antelope with long

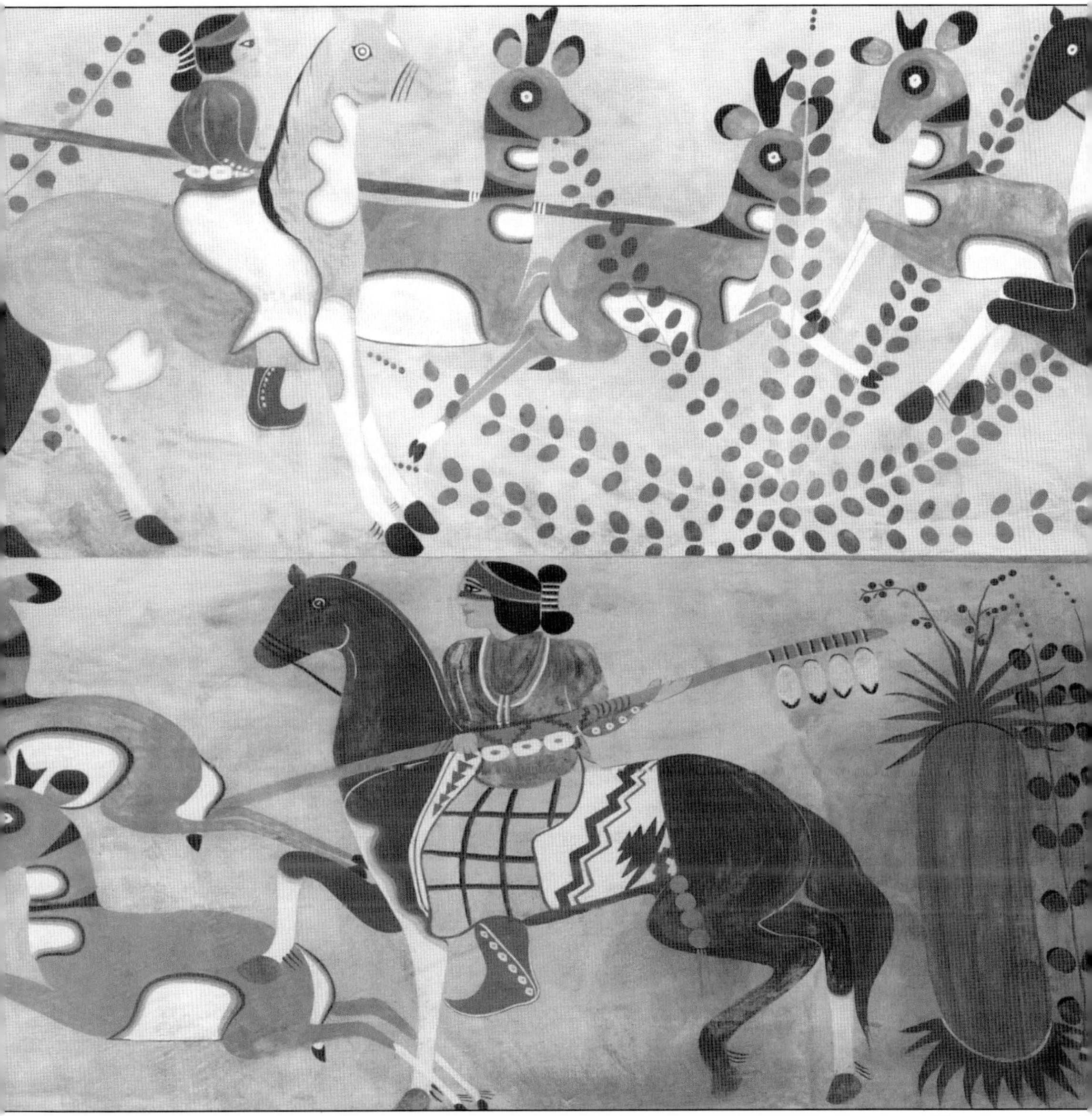

pikes. The plants in the landscape are magnified, as if the viewer is spying near ground level. Narciso worked at a number of occupations besides being an artist, including silversmith, boxer, job placement interviewer, vocational counselor, and interpreter. Much of his painting was done during the 1960s and 1970s. He fathered two children, Tony and Elizabeth, who are also artists. (Courtesy of Skip Maisel.)

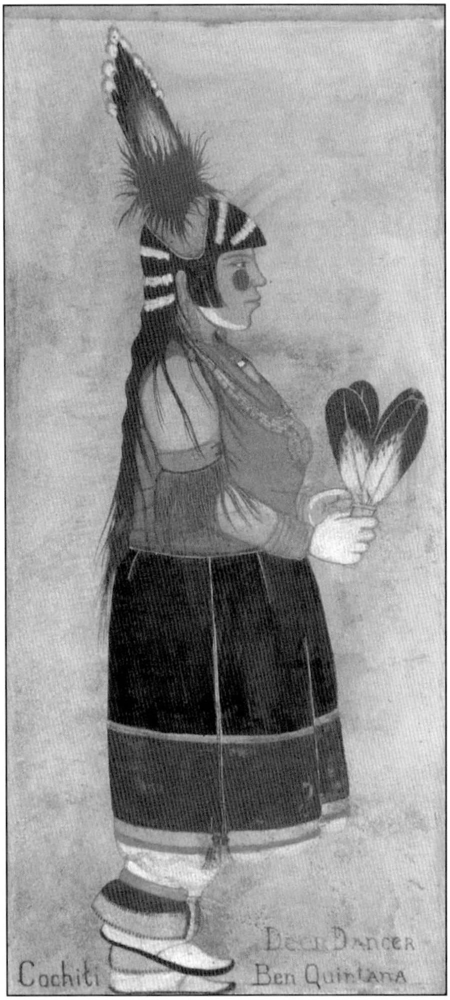

At left, this mural is called *Cochiti Deer Dancer* by Ha A Tee/Ben Quintana, from Cochiti Pueblo (1923–1944). Below is *Cochiti Deer Dancer* (frontal view) by See Ru/Joe H. Herrera, also from Cochiti Pueblo (1923–2001). Here are two views of a female dancer from the same Pueblo. Ha A Tee's is in profile, wearing a simple black dress, and See Ru's frontal view is wearing an embroidered manta. Note that the women deer dancers are quite different from the male deer impersonators depicted on page 121. Cochiti is a Kerasan Pueblo that has a ritual at the end of the performance where "hunters" shoot the dancers with straw arrows and take them home where they are honored as slain game. This is intended to help insure success in an actual hunt. (Both, courtesy of Skip Maisel.)

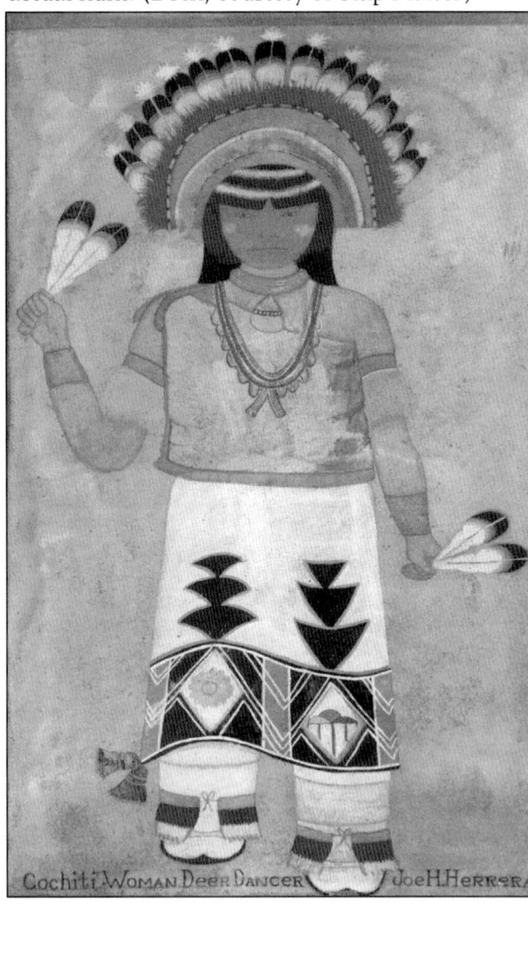

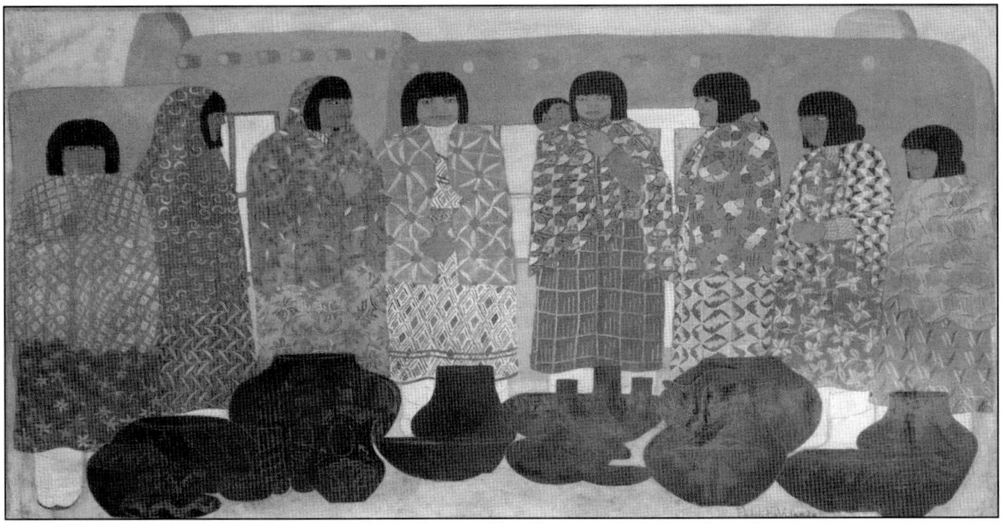

This mural is called *Santa Clara Women Selling Pottery* by Tse Twan (Golden Dawn)/Pablita Velarde, Santa Clara Pueblo (1918–2006). The strong geometric massing of the black pottery in the foreground contrasts with the intricate patterns of the women's clothing. Velarde temporarily lost her sight as a child and it "made me want to see everything. I have trained myself to remember everything I see." Her daughter was famous artist Helen Hardin. (Courtesy of Skip Maisel.)

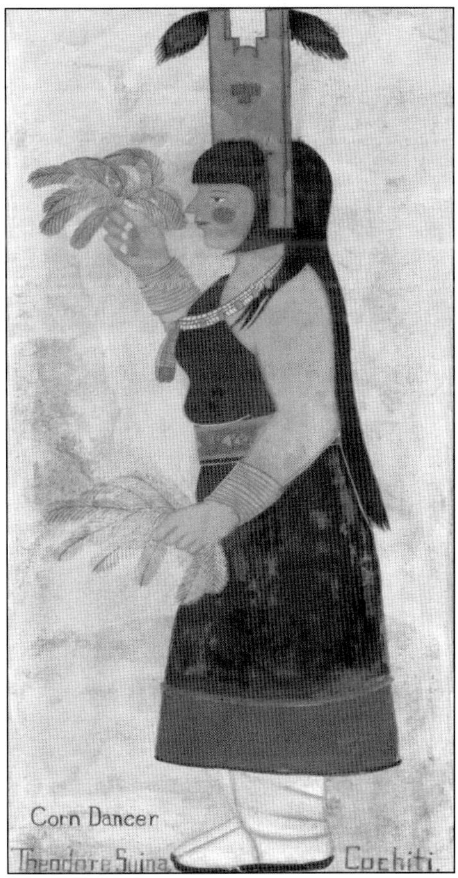

This mural is called *Cochiti Corn Dancer* by Ku-pe-ru (Snow)/Theodore Suina, from Cochiti (1918–present). This corn dancer is interesting to compare with the large corn dance group by Awa Tsireh as well as the single Cochiti deer dancers. Suina served as the governor of Cochiti and worked as a draftsman at Los Alamos Laboratory. He started painting while recovering from a broken neck, the result of a boyhood accident. (Courtesy of Skip Maisel.)

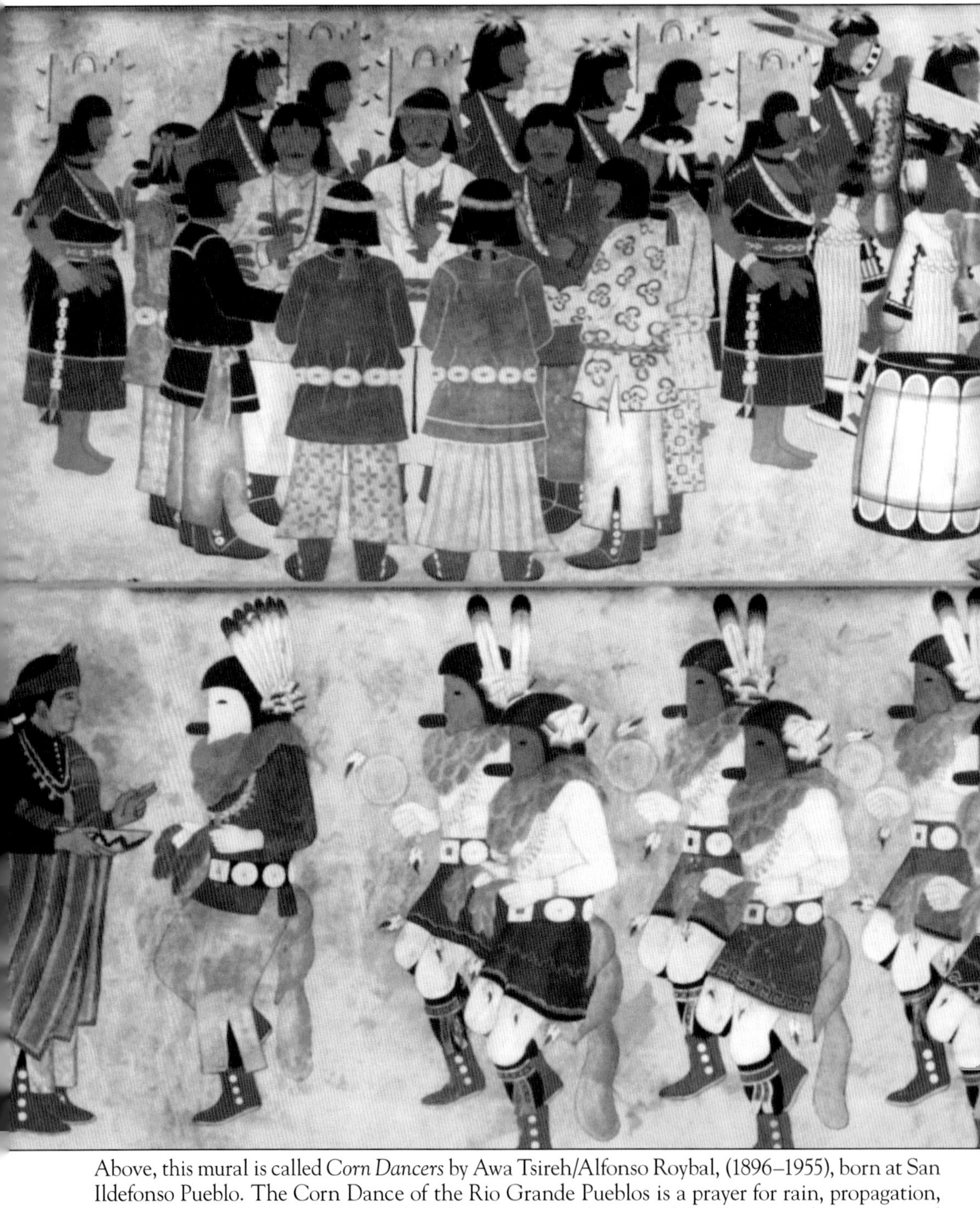

Above, this mural is called *Corn Dancers* by Awa Tsireh/Alfonso Roybal, (1896–1955), born at San Ildefonso Pueblo. The Corn Dance of the Rio Grande Pueblos is a prayer for rain, propagation, and well-being for the Pueblo and for all who attend. The striped figure is a Koshare, or sacred clown. Roybal was an established artist by 1939. Dorothy Dunn wrote of Roybal as he worked on the Maisel mural: "Moving energetically with every stroke, his long braids and bright bandana swinging as he intently followed his pattern. His whole body seemed to emanate assurance and joy

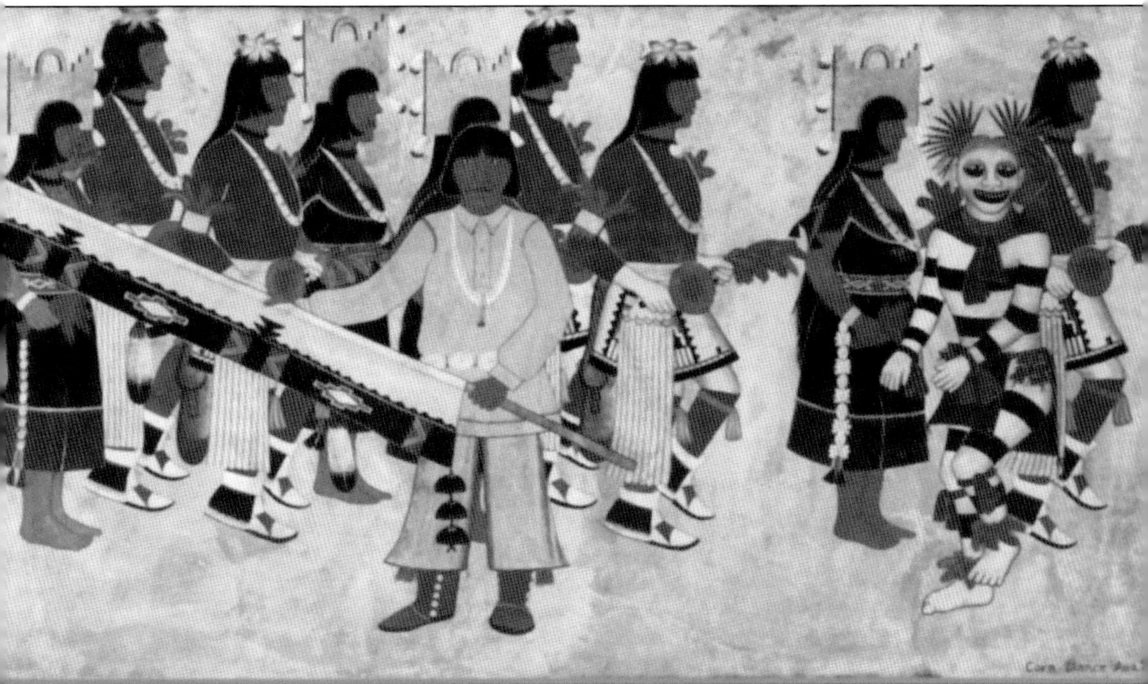

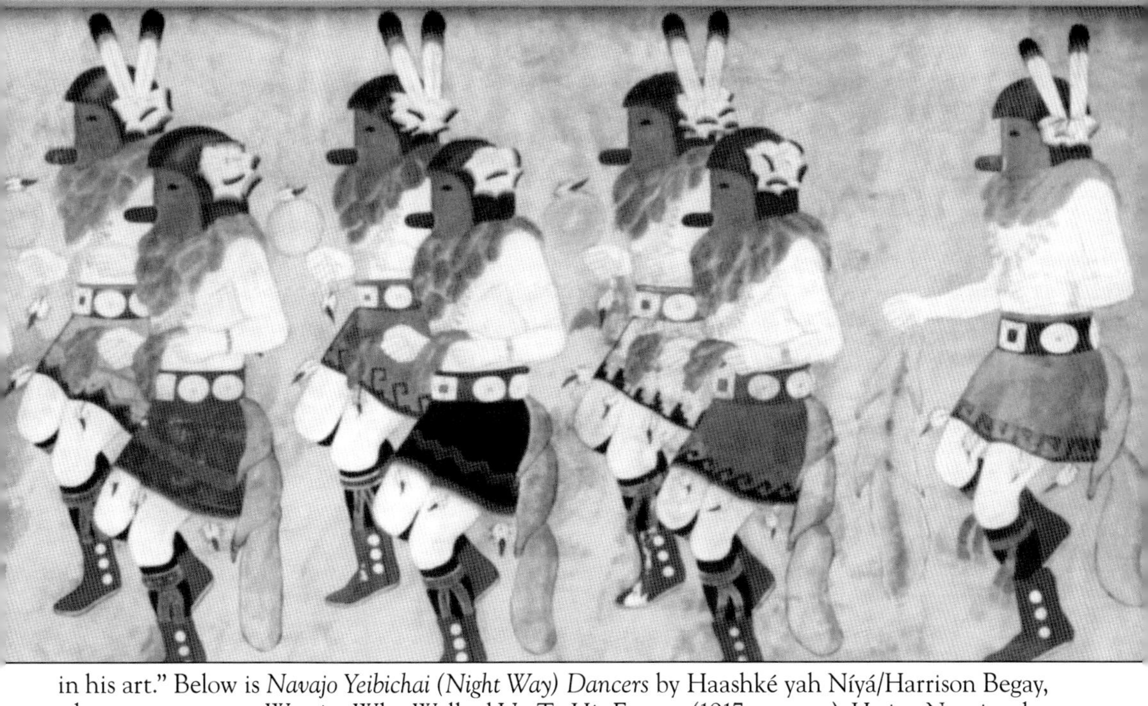

in his art." Below is *Navajo Yeibichai (Night Way) Dancers* by Haashké yah Níyá/Harrison Begay, whose name means Warrior Who Walked Up To His Enemy (1917–present). He is a Navajo who was born in White Cone, Arizona. The Yeibichai is a major winter curing ceremony. Yeis are masked representations of supernatural beings. Begay, now the patriarch of Navajo art, uses fine lines and strong colors with a suggestion of three-dimensional space. (Courtesy of Skip Maisel.)

Consistent with our mission to preserve history on a local level, this book was printed in South Carolina on American-made paper and manufactured entirely in the United States. Products carrying the accredited Forest Stewardship Council (FSC) label are printed on 100 percent FSC-certified paper.